A FEAST OF INFORMATION—
for people who love to eat but need to know
the calorie count of their meals.

THE BARBARA KRAUS 1984 CALORIE
GUIDE TO BRAND NAMES & BASIC FOODS
lists thousands of basic and ready-to-eat foods
from appetizers to desserts—carry it to the
supermarket, to the restaurant, to the beach, to
the coffee cart, and on trips.

Flip through these fact-filled pages. Mix, match,
and keep track of calories as they add up. But
remember, strawberry shortcake is fattening any
way you slice it!

The Barbara Kraus
1984 Calorie
Guide to
Brand Names and
Basic Foods

SIGNET Books by Barbara Kraus

The Barbara Kraus 1984 Calorie Guide to Brand Names and Basic Foods

A SIGNET BOOK

NEW AMERICAN LIBRARY

Copyright © 1971, 1973, 1975, 1976, 1977 by Barbara Kraus.
© 1978 by John R. Fernbach, Esq. and Murray Cohen,
Co-Executors to the Estate of Barbara Kraus.
Copyright © 1979, 1980, 1981, 1982, 1983 by The New American Library, Inc.

Excerpted from *Dictionary of Calories and Carbohydrates*

SIGNET TRADEMARK REG. U.S. PAT. OFF. AND FOREIGN COUNTRIES
REGISTERED TRADEMARK—MARCA REGISTRADA
HECHO EN CHICAGO, U.S.A.

SIGNET, SIGNET CLASSIC, MENTOR, PLUME, MERIDIAN and NAL BOOKS
are published by The New American Library, Inc.,
1633 Broadway, New York, New York 10019

FIRST PRINTING, JANUARY, 1984

1 2 3 4 5 6 7 8 9

PRINTED IN THE UNITED STATES OF AMERICA

For Joe, Pam, Kim,
and Joey Cristodaro

Foreword

The composition of the foods we eat is not static: it changes from time to time. In the case of *brand-name* products, manufacturers alter their recipes to reflect the availability of ingredients, advances in technology, or improvements in formulae. Each year new products appear on the market and some old ones are discontinued.

On the other hand, information on *basic foods* such as meats, vegetables, and fruits may also change as a result of the development of better analytical methods, different growing conditions, or new marketing practices. These changes, however, are usually relatively small as compared with those in manufactured products.

Some differences may be found between the values in this book and those appearing on the product labels. This is usually due to the fact that the Food and Drug Administration permits manufacturers to round the figures reported on labels. The data in this book are reported as calculated without rounding. If large differences between the two sets of values are noted, they may be due to changes in product formulae, and in those cases the label data should be used.

For all these reasons, a book of calorie or nutritive values of foods must be kept up to date by a periodic reviewing and revision of the data presented.

Therefore, this handy calorie counter will provide each year the most current and accurate estimates available. Generous use of this little book will help you and your family to select the right foods and the proper number of calories each member requires to gain, lose, or maintain healthy and attractive weight.

Good eating in 1984! For 1985, we'll pick up the new products, drop any has-beens, and make whatever other changes are necessary.

Barbara Kraus

Why This Book?

Some of the data presented here can be found in more detail in my best-selling *Calories and Carbohydrates*, a dictionary of 8,000 brand names and basic foods. Complete as it is, it is meant to be used as a reference book at home or in the office and not to be squeezed into a suit jacket or evening bag—it's just too big.

Therefore, responding to the need for a portable calorie guide, and one which can reflect food changes often, I have written this smaller and handier version. The selection of material and the additional new entries provide readers with pertinent data on thousands of products that they would prepare at home to take to work, eat in a restaurant or luncheonette, nibble on from the coffee cart, take to the beach, buy in the candy store, etcetera.

For the sake of saving space and providing you with a greater selection of products, I had to make certain compromises: whereas in the giant book there are several physical descriptions of a product, here there is but one.

For Beginners Only

The language of dieting is no more difficult to learn than any other new subject; in many respects, it's much easier, particularly if you restrict your education to clearly defined goals.

For you who never before had the need or the interest in a lesson in weight control, I offer the following elementary introduction, applicable to any diet, self-initiated or suggested by your doctor, nutritionist, or dietician.

A Calorie

An analysis of foods in terms of calories is most often the chosen method to describe the relative energy yielded by foods.

A calorie is a shorthand way to summarize the units of energy contained in any foodstuff or alcoholic beverage, similar to the way a thermometer indicates heat. One pound of fat is equal to 3,500 calories. Add this number of calories to those you need to balance your energy requirements and you will gain one pound; subtract it and you will lose a pound.

Other Nutrients

Carbohydrates—which include sugars, starches, and acids—are only one of several chemical compounds in foods that yield calories. Proteins, found mainly in beef, poultry, and fish; fats, found in oils, butter, marbling of meat, poultry skin; and alcohol, found in some beverages, also contribute calories. Except for alcohol, most foods contain at least some of these nutrients:

The amount of carbohydrates varies from zero in meats and a trace in alcohol to a heavy concentration in sugar, syrups, some fruits, grains, and root vegetables.

As of this date, the most respected nutritional researchers insist that some carbohydrate is necessary every day for maintaining good health. The amount to be included is an individual matter, and in any drastic effort to change your eating patterns, be sure to consult your doctor first.

Now, on how to use this new language.

To begin with, you use this book like a dictionary. If your plan is to cut down on calories, the easiest way to do so is to consult the portable calorie counter and keep an accurate count of your total intake of food and beverages for a period of seven days. If you have not gained or lost weight during that week, divide that number by seven and you'll have your maintenance diet expressed in calories. To lose weight, you must reduce your daily or weekly intake of calories below this maintenance level. (To gain, increase the intake.)

Keeping in mind that you want to stay healthy and eat well-balanced meals (which include the basic food groups: milk or milk products; meat, poultry, or fish; vegetables and fruits; and whole grain or enriched breads or cereals, as well as some fats or oils), you then start to cut down on your portion in order to reduce your intake of calories. There are many imaginative ways to diet without total withdrawal from one's favorite foods.

Once you know and don't have to guess what calories are in your foods, you can relax and enjoy it. It could turn out that dieting isn't so bad after all.

ABBREVIATIONS AND SYMBOLS

* = prepared as package directs[1]
< = less than
& = and
" = inch
canned = bottles or jars as well as cans
dia. = diameter
fl. = fluid
liq. = liquid
lb. = pound
med. = medium

oz. = ounce
pkg. = package
pt. = pint
qt. = quart
sq. = square
T. = tablespoon
Tr. = trace
tsp. = teaspoon
wt. = weight

Italics or name in parentheses = registered trademark, ®. All data not identified by company or trademark are based on material obtained from the United States Department of Agriculture or Health, Education and Welfare/Food and Agriculture Organization.

EQUIVALENTS

By Weight	By Volume
1 pound = 16 ounces	1 quart = 4 cups
1 ounce = 28.35 grams	1 cup = 8 fluid ounces
3.52 ounces = 100 grams	1 cup = ½ pint
	1 cup = 16 tablespoons
	2 tablespoons = 1 fluid ounce
	1 tablespoon = 3 teaspoons
	1 pound butter = 4 sticks or 2 cups

[1]If the package directions call for whole or skim milk, the data given here are for whole milk unless otherwise stated.

Food and Description	Measure or Quantity	Calories

A

ABALONE, canned	4 oz.	91
AC'CENT	¼ tsp.	3
ACEROLA, fresh, fruit	4 oz.	32
ALBACORE, raw, meat only	4 oz.	201
ALEXANDER COCKTAIL MIX		
(Holland House)	1 serving	69
ALLSPICE (French's)	1 tsp.	6
ALMOND:		
In shell	10 nuts	60
Shelled, raw, natural with skins	1 oz.	170
Roasted, dry (Planters)	1 oz.	170
Roasted, oil (Fisher)	1 oz.	178
ALMOND EXTRACT:		
(Durkee) pure	1 tsp.	13
(Virginia Dare) 34% alcohol	1 tsp.	10
ALPHA-BITS, cereal (Post)	1 cup (1 oz.)	113
AMARETTO DI SARONNO	1 fl. oz.	82
A. M. FRUIT DRINK (Mott's)	6 fl. oz.	90
ANCHOVY, PICKLED, canned, flat or rolled, not heavily salted, drained	2-oz. can	79
ANISE EXTRACT (Durkee) imitation	1 tsp.	16
ANISE SEED, dried	½ oz.	58
ANISETTE:		
(DeKuyper)	1 fl. oz.	95
(Mr. Boston)	1 fl. oz.	88
APPLE:		
Eaten with skin	2½" dia.	66
Eaten without skin	2½" dia.	53
Canned (Comstock):		
Rings, drained	1 ring	30
Sliced	⅙ of 21-oz. can	45
Dried:		
(Del Monte)	1 cup	151
(Sun-Maid)	2-oz. serving	150
Frozen, sweetened	10-oz. pkg.	264
APPLE BROWN BETTY	1 cup	325
APPLE BUTTER (Smucker's) cider	1 T.	38
APPLE-CHERRY JUICE, Cocktail, canned, *Musselman's*	8 fl. oz.	110
APPLE CIDER:		
Canned (Mott's) sweet	½ cup	59
Mix, Country Time	8 fl. oz.	98

1

Food and Description	Measure or Quantity	Calories
APPLE-CRANBERRY DRINK		
(Hi-C):		
Canned	6 fl. oz.	90
*Mix	6 fl. oz.	72
APPLE-CRANBERRY JUICE,		
canned (Lincoln)	6 fl. oz.	100
APPLE DRINK:		
Canned:		
Capri Sun, natural	6¾ fl. oz.	90
(Hi-C)	6 fl. oz.	92
*Mix (Hi-C)	6 fl. oz.	72
APPLE DUMPLINGS, frozen		
(Pepperidge Farm)	1 dumpling	260
APPLE, ESCALLOPED, frozen		
(Stouffer's)	4 oz.	138
APPLE-GRAPE JUICE, canned:		
Musselman's	6 fl. oz.	82
(Red Cheek)	6 fl. oz.	69
APPLE JACKS, cereal (Kellogg's)	1 cup (1 oz.)	110
APPLE JAM (Smucker's)	1 T.	53
APPLE JELLY:		
Sweetened (Smucker's)	1 T.	67
Dietetic (See APPLE SPREAD)		
APPLE JUICE:		
Canned:		
(Lincoln)	6 fl. oz.	96
(Minute Maid)	6 fl. oz.	100
(Mott's)	6 fl. oz.	80
Musselman's	6 fl. oz.	80
(Red Cheek)	6 fl. oz.	83
(Seneca Foods)	6 fl. oz.	90
Chilled (Minute Maid)	6 fl. oz.	100
*Frozen:		
(Minute Maid)	6 fl. oz.	100
(Seneca Foods) Vitamin C added	6 fl. oz.	90
(Seneca Foods) natural style,		
Vitamin C added	6 fl. oz.	84
APPLE PIE (See PIE, Apple)		
APPLE SAUCE:		
Regular:		
(Del Monte)	½ cup	96
(Mott's):		
Natural	½ cup	115
With ground cranberries	½ cup	110
Musselman's	½ cup	96
(Stokely-Van Camp)	½ cup	90
Dietetic:		
(Diet Delight)	½ cup	50

Food and Description	Measure or Quantity	Calories
(Featherweight) water pack	½ cup	50
(Mott's) natural	4-oz. serving	50
Musselman's, natural	½ cup	50
(Seneca Foods) 100% natural	½ cup	50
(S&W) *Nutradiet*	½ cup	55
APPLE SPREAD, low sugar:		
(Dia-Mel)	1 T.	6
(Diet Delight)	1 T.	12
(Featherweight):		
Regular	1 T.	16
Artificially sweetened	1 T.	6
(Slenderella)	1 T.	24
(Smucker's)	1 T.	24
(Tillie Lewis) *Tasti Diet*	1 T.	12
APPLE STRUDEL, frozen		
(Pepperidge Farm)	3-oz. serving	240
APRICOT:		
Fresh, whole	1 apricot	18
Canned, regular pack:		
(Del Monte) whole, peeled	1 cup	220
(Libby's) halves, heavy syrup	1 cup	221
(Stokely-Van Camp)	1 cup	220
Canned, dietetic:		
(Del Monte) *Lite*	½ cup	64
(Diet Delight):		
Syrup pack	½ cup	60
Water pack	½ cup	35
(Featherweight):		
Juice pack	½ cup	50
Water pack	½ cup	35
(Libby's) Lite	½ cup	60
(S&W) *Nutradiet*:		
Halves, juice pack	½ cup	50
Halves, water pack	½ cup	35
Whole, juice pack	½ cup	40
Dried:		
(Del Monte)	2-oz. serving	150
(Sun-Maid; Sunsweet)	¼ cup (1.7 oz.)	125
APRICOT LIQUEUR (DeKuyper)	1 fl. oz.	82
APRICOT NECTAR:		
(Del Monte)	6 fl. oz.	113
(Libby's)	6 fl. oz.	110
APRICOT-PINEAPPLE NECTAR, canned, dietetic (S&W) *Nutradiet*	6-oz. serving	35
APRICOT & PINEAPPLE PRESERVE OR JAM:		
Sweetened (Smucker's)	1 T.	53

Food and Description	Measure or Quantity	Calories
Dietetic (See APRICOT & PINEAPPLE SPREAD)		
APRICOT-PINEAPPLE SPREAD, low sugar:		
(Diet Delight)	1 T.	6
(Featherweight) artificially sweetened	1 T.	6
(S&W) *Nutradiet*	1 T.	12
(Tillie Lewis) *Tasti Diet*	1 T.	12
APRICOT SOUR COCKTAIL (National Distillers-*Duet*)		
12½% alcohol	2 fl. oz.	48
ARBY'S:		
Beef & Cheese Sandwich	6 oz.	450
Club Sandwich	9 oz.	560
Ham 'N Cheese	5½ oz.	380
Roast Beef:		
Regular	5 oz.	350
Junior	3 oz.	220
Super	9¾ oz.	620
Turkey Deluxe	8½ oz.	510
ARTICHOKE:		
Boiled	15-oz. artichoke	187
Canned (Cara Mia) marinated, drained	6-oz. jar	175
Frozen:		
(Birds Eye) deluxe, hearts	⅓ pkg.	39
(Cara Mia)	3-oz. serving	35
ASPARAGUS:		
Boiled	1 spear (½″ dia. at base)	3
Canned, regular pack, spears, solids & liq.:		
(Del Monte) green or white	1 cup	44
(Festal) green or white	1 cup	48
(Green Giant) green	8-oz. can	46
Musselman's	1 cup	40
(Stokely-Van Camp)	1 cup	45
Canned, dietetic, solids & liq.:		
(Diet Delight)	½ cup	16
(Featherweight) cut spears	1 cup	40
(S&W) *Nutradiet*	1 cup	40
Frozen:		
(Birds Eye):		
Cuts	⅓ pkg.	29
Spears, regular or jumbo deluxe	⅓ pkg.	30
(Green Giant) cuts, butter sauce	3 oz.	57
(McKenzie)	⅓ pkg.	25
(Seabrook Farms)	⅓ pkg.	30

4

Food and Description	Measure or Quantity	Calories
(Stouffer's) souffle	⅓ pkg.	118
AUNT JEMIMA SYRUP		
(See SYRUP)		
AVOCADO, all varieties	1 fruit	378
***AWAKE** (Birds Eye)	6 fl. oz.	91
AYDS:		
Butterscotch	1 piece	27
Chocolate, chocolate mint, vanilla	1 piece	26

B

Food and Description	Measure or Quantity	Calories
BACON, broiled (Oscar Mayer):		
Regular slice	6-gram slice	35
Thick slice	1 slice	64
BACON BITS:		
(Betty Crocker) *Bac*Os*	1 tsp.	13
(Durkee) imitation	1 tsp.	8
(French's) imitation	1 tsp.	6
(Libby's) crumbles	1 tsp.	8
(Oscar Mayer) real	1 tsp.	6
BACON, CANADIAN, unheated:		
(Hormel) sliced	1-oz. serving	50
(Oscar Mayer) 93% fat free	.7-oz. slice	30
(Oscar Mayer) 93% fat free	1-oz. slice	40
BACON, SIMULATED, cooked:		
(Oscar Mayer) *Lean 'N Tasty:*		
Beef	1 slice	39
Pork	1 slice	45
(Swift) *Sizzlean*	1 strip	50
BAGEL:		
Egg	3-inch diameter, 1.9 oz.	162
Water	3-inch diameter, 1.9 oz.	163
BAKING POWDER:		
(Calumet)	1 tsp.	7
(Featherweight) low sodium, cereal free	1 tsp.	8
BAMBOO SHOOTS:		
Raw, trimmed	¼ lb.	31
Canned, drained:		
(Chun King)	½ of 8½-oz. can	20
(La Choy)	½ cup	12
BANANA, medium	6.3-oz. banana (weighed unpeeled)	101

Food and Description	Measure or Quantity	Calories
BANANA EXTRACT (Durkee)		
imitation	1 tsp.	15
BANANA PIE (See PIE, Banana)		
BARBECUE SEASONING (French's)	1 tsp.	6
BARDOLINO WINE (Antinori)	1 fl. oz.	28
BARLEY, pearled (Quaker Scotch)	¼ cup	172
BASIL (French's)	1 tsp.	3
BASS:		
Baked, stuffed	3½ " × 4½" × 1½"	531
Oven-fried	8¾" × 4½" × ⅝"	392
BAY LEAF (French's)	1 tsp.	5
B & B LIQUEUR	1 fl. oz.	94
B.B.Q. SAUCE & BEEF, frozen		
(Banquet) *Cookin' Bag*, sliced	5-oz. cooking bag	126
BEAN, BAKED:		
(USDA):		
With pork & molasses sauce	1 cup	382
With pork & tomato sauce	1 cup	311
Canned:		
(B&M):		
Pea bean with pork in brown sugar sauce	8 oz.	330
Red kidney bean in brown sugar sauce	8 oz.	330
(Campbell):		
Home style	8-oz. can	270
With pork & tomato sauce	8-oz. can	270
(Grandma Brown's)	8-oz. serving	289
(Libby's):		
Deep Brown, with pork & molasses sauce	½ of 14-oz. can	228
Deep Brown, vegetarian in tomato sauce	½ of 14-oz. can	214
(Sultana) with pork & tomato sauce	½ of 16-oz. can	232
(Van Camp) with pork	8 oz.	226
BEAN, BARBECUE (Campbell)	7⅞-oz. can	250
BEAN, BLACK, DRY	1 cup	678
BEAN, BROWN, DRY	1 cup	678
BEAN & FRANKFURTER, canned:		
(Campbell) in tomato and molasses sauce	8-oz. can	350
(Hormel) *Short Orders*, 'n wieners	7½-oz. can	290
BEAN & FRANKFURTER DINNER, frozen:		
(Banquet)	10¾-oz. dinner	591
(Swanson) *TV Brand*	11¼-oz. dinner	490
BEAN, GARBANZO, canned, dietetic (S&W) *Nutradiet*, low sodium	½ cup	105

Food and Description	Measure or Quantity	Calories
BEAN, GREEN:		
Boiled, 1½" to 2" pieces, drained	½ cup	17
Canned, regular pack:		
(Comstock) solids & liq.	½ cup	23
(Del Monte) French, drained	½ cup	27
(Green Giant) French or whole, solids & liq.	½ of 8½-oz. can	21
(Libby's) French, solids & liq.	½ cup	21
(Stokely-Van Camp) solids & liq.	½ cup	20
(Sunshine) solids & liq.	½ cup	20
Canned, dietetic:		
(Diet Delight) solids & liq.	½ cup	20
(Featherweight) cut or French, solids & liq.	½ cup	25
(S&W) *Nutradiet*, cut, solids & liq., low sodium	½ cup	20
Frozen:		
(Birds Eye):		
Cut	⅓ pkg.	30
French, with mushrooms	⅓ pkg.	34
Italian style	⅓ pkg.	38
Whole, deluxe	⅓ pkg.	26
(Green Giant):		
With butter sauce	⅓ pkg.	34
With mushroom in cream sauce	⅓ pkg.	66
(McKenzie) cut or french style	⅓ pkg.	25
(Seabrook Farms)	⅓ pkg.	29
(Southland) cut or french style	⅕ of 16-oz. pkg.	25
BEAN, GREEN, & MUSHROOM CASSEROLE		
(Stouffer's)	½ pkg.	143
BEAN, GREEN, WITH POTATOES, canned (Sunshine) solids & liq.	½ cup	34
BEAN, GREEN, PUREE, canned, dietetic (Featherweight)	1 cup	70
BEAN, ITALIAN:		
Canned (Del Monte) drained	½ cup	43
Frozen (McKenzie; Seabrook Farms)	⅓ pkg.	37
BEAN, KIDNEY:		
Canned, regular pack:		
(Furman) red, fancy, light	½ cup	121
(Van Camp):		
Light	8 oz.	194
New Orleans style	8 oz.	188
Red	8 oz.	213
Canned, dietetic (S&W) *Nutradiet*, low sodium, solids & liq.	½ cup	90

7

Food and Description	Measure or Quantity	Calories
BEAN, LIMA:		
Boiled, drained	½ cup	94
Canned, regular pack:		
(Del Monte) drained	½ cup	107
(Libby's) solids & liq.	½ cup	91
(Sultana) butter bean	¼ of 15-oz. can	82
Canned, dietetic (Featherweight) solids & liq.	½ cup	80
Frozen:		
(Birds Eye) tiny, deluxe	⅓ pkg.	111
(Green Giant):		
In butter sauce	3 oz.	93
Harvest Fresh	4 oz.	180
(McKenzie):		
Baby Lima	⅓ pkg.	130
Fordhook	⅓ pkg.	100
Tiny	⅓ pkg.	110
(Seabrook Farms):		
Baby Lima	⅓ pkg.	126
Baby butter bean	⅓ pkg.	139
Fordhooks	⅓ pkg.	98
BEAN, PINTO (Del Monte) spicy	½ cup	120
BEAN, REFRIED, canned:		
(Del Monte) regular or spicy	½ cup	130
Old El Paso	½ of 8¼-oz. can	103
(Ortega) lightly spicy or true bean	½ cup	170
BEAN SALAD, canned:		
(Green Giant)	4¼-oz. serving	91
(Nalley's)	4½-oz. serving	155
BEAN SOUP (See SOUP, Bean)		
BEAN SPROUT:		
Mung, raw	½ lb.	80
Mung, boiled, drained	¼ lb.	32
Soy, raw	½ lb.	104
Soy, boiled, drained	¼ lb.	43
Canned:		
(Chun King) drained	8 oz.	40
(La Choy) drained	⅔ cup	7
BEAN, YELLOW OR WAX:		
Broiled, 1" pieces, drained	½ cup	18
Canned, regular pack:		
(Comstock) solids & liq.	½ cup	22
(Del Monte) cut, solids & liq.	½ cup	18
(Festal) cut or French style, solids & liq.	½ cup	19
(Libby's) cut, solids & liq.	4 oz.	23
(Stokely-Van Camp) solids & liq.	½ cup	23

Food and Description	Measure or Quantity	Calories
Canned, dietetic (Featherweight, cut, solids & liq.)	½ cup	25
Frozen (McKenzie) cut	⅓ pkg.	25
BEEF, choice grade, medium done:		
Brisket, braised:		
Lean & fat	3 oz.	350
Lean only	3 oz.	189
Chuck, pot roast:		
Lean & fat	3 oz.	278
Lean only	3 oz.	182
Fat, separable, cooked	1 oz.	207
Filet Mignon. See Steak, sirloin, lean		
Flank, braised, 100% lean	3 oz.	167
Ground:		
Regular, raw	½ cup	303
Regular, broiled	3 oz.	243
Lean, broiled	3 oz.	186
Rib:		
Roasted, lean & fat	3 oz.	374
Lean only	3 oz.	205
Round:		
Broiled, lean & fat	3 oz.	222
Lean only	3 oz.	161
Rump:		
Roasted, lean & fat	3 oz.	295
Lean only	3 oz.	177
Steak, club, broiled:		
One 8-oz. steak (weighed without bone before cooking) will give you:		
Lean & fat	5.9 oz.	754
Lean only	3.4 oz.	234
Steak, porterhouse, broiled:		
One 16-oz. steak (weighed with bone before cooking) will give you:		
Lean & fat	10.2 oz.	1339
Lean only	5.9 oz.	372
Steak, ribeye, broiled:		
One 10-oz. steak (weighed without bone before cooking) will give you:		
Lean & fat	7.3 oz.	911
Lean only	3.8 oz.	258
Steak, sirloin, double-bone, broiled:		
One 16-oz. steak (weighed with bone before cooking) will give you:		

Food and Description	Measure or Quantity	Calories
Lean & fat	8.9 oz.	1028
Lean only	5.9 oz.	359
One 12-oz. steak (weighed with bone before cooking) will give you:		
Lean & fat	6.6 oz.	767
Lean only	4.4 oz.	268
Steak, T-bone, broiled:		
One 16-oz. steak (weighed with bone before cooking) will give you:		
Lean & fat	9.8 oz.	1315
Lean only	5.5 oz.	348
BEEFAMATO COCKTAIL (Mott's)	6 fl. oz.	70
BEEF BOUILLON:		
(Herb-Ox):		
Cube	1 cube	6
Packet	1 packet	8
MBT	1 packet	14
Low sodium (Featherweight)	1 tsp.	18
BEEF, CHIPPED:		
Cooked, home recipe	½ cup	188
Frozen:		
(Banquet) creamed, *Cookin' Bag*	5-oz. pkg.	124
(Stouffer's) creamed	5½-oz.	231
(Swanson) creamed	10½-oz. entree	330
BEEF DINNER or ENTREE, frozen:		
(Banquet):		
Regular	11-oz. dinner	312
Chopped	11-oz. dinner	443
Man Pleaser, sliced	20-oz. dinner	453
(Morton):		
Regular	10-oz. dinner	261
Country Table, sliced	14-oz. dinner	512
Steak House, sirloin strip	9½-oz. dinner	896
(Swanson):		
Hungry Man, chopped	18-oz. dinner	690
Hungry Man, sliced	12¼-oz. entree	300
TV Brand, chopped sirloin	10-oz. dinner	380
3-course	15-oz. dinner	450
(Weight Watchers):		
Beefsteak, 2-compartment meal	9¾-oz. pkg.	344
Sirloin in mushroom sauce, 3-compartment meal	13-oz. pkg.	410
BEEF, DRIED, canned:		
(Hormel) *Short Orders,* creamed	7½-oz. can	160
(Swift)	1-oz. serving	47

Food and Description	Measure or Quantity	Calories
BEEF GOULASH (Hormel)		
Short Orders	7½-oz. can	230
BEEF, GROUND, SEASONING MIX:		
*(Durkee):		
Regular	1 cup	653
With onion	1 cup	659
(French's) with onion	1⅛-oz. pkg.	100
BEEF HASH, ROAST:		
Canned, *Mary Kitchen*:		
Regular	7½-oz. serving	396
Short Orders	7½-oz. can	370
Frozen (Stouffer's)	½ of 11½-oz. serving	262
BEEF PEPPER ORIENTAL:		
*Canned (La Choy):		
Regular	¾ cup	90
Bi-pack	¾ cup	70
Frozen (Chun King):		
Dinner	11-oz. dinner	310
Pouch	6-oz. serving	80
BEEF PIE, frozen:		
(Banquet):		
Regular	8-oz. pie	409
Supreme	8 oz. pie	380
(Morton)	8-oz. pie	316
(Swanson):		
Regular	8-oz. pie	400
Hungry-Man	16-oz. pie	720
BEEF PUFFS, frozen (Durkee)	1 piece	47
BEEF, SHORT RIBS, frozen (Stouffer's) boneless, with vegetable gravy	½ of 11½-oz. pkg.	347
BEEF SOUP (See SOUP, Beef)		
BEEF SPREAD, ROAST, canned (Underwood)	½ of 4¾-oz. can	140
BEEF STEW:		
Home recipe, made with lean beef chuck	1 cup	218
Canned, regular pack:		
Dinty Moore:		
Regular	7½-oz. serving	184
Short Orders	7½-oz. can	170
(Libby's)	½ of 15-oz. can	160
(Nalley's)	7½-oz. serving	226
(Swanson)	7⅝-oz. serving	150
Canned, dietetic (Featherweight)	7½-oz. serving	220
Frozen:		
(Banquet) *Buffet Supper*	2-lb. pkg.	700

11

Food and Description	Measure or Quantity	Calories
(Green Giant):		
Boil 'N Bag	9-oz. entree	178
Twin pouch, with noodles	9-oz. entree	333
(Stouffer's)	10-oz. serving	305
BEEF STEW SEASONING MIX:		
*(Durkee)	1 cup	379
(French's)	1 pkg.	150
BEEF STOCK BASE (French's)	1 tsp.	8
BEEF STIX (Vienna)	1 oz.	163
BEEF STROGANOFF, frozen		
(Stouffer's) with parsley noodles	9¾ oz.	390
*BEEF STROGANOFF SEASONING		
MIX (Durkee)	1 cup	820
BEER & ALE:		
Regular:		
Black Horse Ale	8 fl. oz.	108
Budweiser	8 fl. oz.	100
Busch Bavarian	8 fl. oz.	100
Michelob	8 fl. oz.	113
Pearl Premium	8 fl. oz.	99
Stroh Bohemian, regular	8 fl. oz.	99
Stroh Bohemian, 3.2 low gravity	8 fl. oz.	84
Tuborg, USA	8 fl. oz.	93
Light or low carbohydrate:		
Budweiser Light	8 fl. oz.	75
Gablinger's	8 fl. oz.	66
Michelob, light	8 fl. oz.	90
Natural Light	8 fl. oz.	75
Pearl Lite	12 fl. oz.	68
Stroh Light	8 fl. oz.	77
BEER, NEAR:		
Goetz Pale	8 fl. oz.	53
Kingsbury (Heileman)	8 fl. oz.	30
(Metbrew)	8 fl. oz.	49
BEET:		
Boiled, whole	2″ dia. beet	16
Boiled, sliced	½ cup	33
Canned, regular pack:		
(Del Monte):		
Pickled, solids & liq.	4 oz.	77
Sliced, solids & liq.	4 oz.	29
(Greenwood):		
Harvard, solids & liq.	½ cup	70
Pickled, solids & liq.	½ cup	110
Pickled, with onion, solids & liq.	½ cup	115
(Libby's) Harvard, solids & liq.	½ cup	87
(Stokely-Van Camp) pickled, solids & liq.	½ cup	95

Food and Description	Measure or Quantity	Calories
Canned, dietetic:		
(Blue Boy) whole, solids & liq.	½ cup	39
(Comstock) solids & liq.	½ cup	30
(Featherweight) sliced, solids & liq.	½ cup	45
(S&W) *Nutradiet,* sliced, solids & liq.	½ cup	35
BEET PUREE, canned, dietetic (Featherweight)	1 cup	90
BENEDICTINE LIQUEUR (Julius Wile)	1½ fl. oz.	168
BIG H, burger sauce (Hellmann's)	1 T.	71
BIG MAC (See McDONALD's)		
BIG WHEEL (Hostess)	1 piece	172
BISCUIT DOUGH (Pillsbury):		
Baking Powder, *1969 Brand*	1 biscuit	100
Big Country	1 biscuit	95
Big Country, Good 'N Buttery	1 biscuit	100
Buttermilk:		
Regular	1 biscuit	50
Ballard, Oven Ready	1 biscuit	50
Extra Lights	1 biscuit	60
Extra rich, *Hungry Jack*	1 biscuit	65
Fluffy, *Hungry Jack*	1 biscuit	100
Butter Tastin', 1869 Brand	1 biscuit	100
Butter Tastin', Hungry Jack	1 biscuit	95
Dinner	1 biscuit	55
Flaky, *Hungry Jack*	1 biscuit	90
Oven Ready, Ballard	1 biscuit	50
BITTERS (Angostura)	1 tsp.	14
BLACKBERRY, fresh, hulled	1 cup	84
BLACKBERRY JELLY:		
Sweetened (Smucker's)	1 T.	53
Dietetic (See BLACKBERRY SPREAD)		
BLACKBERRY LIQUEUR (Bols)	1 fl. oz.	95
BLACKBERRY PRESERVE OR JAM:		
Sweetened (Smucker's)	1 T.	53
Dietetic:		
(Dia-Mel)	1 T.	6
(Diet-Delight)	1 T.	12
(Featherweight)	1 T.	16
(S&W) *Nutradiet*	1 T.	12
BLACKBERRY SPREAD, low sugar:		
(Diet Delight)	1 T.	12
(Featherweight)	1 T.	16
(Smucker's)	1 T.	24

Food and Description	Measure or Quantity	Calories
BLACKBERRY WINE		
(Mogen David)	3 fl. oz.	135
BLACK-EYED PEAS:		
Canned:		
(Sultana) with pork	7½-oz. serving	204
(Sunshine) with pork, solids & liq.	½ cup	90
Frozen:		
(McKenzie)	⅓ pkg.	130
(Seabrook Farms)	⅓ pkg.	130
(Southland)	⅕ of 16-oz. pkg.	120
BLINTZE, frozen (King Kold) cheese	2½-oz. piece	132
BLOODY MARY MIX:		
Dry (Bar-Tender's)	1 serving	26
Liquid (Sacramento)	5½-fl. oz. can	39
BLUEBERRY, fresh, whole	½ cup	45
BLUEBERRY PIE (See PIE, Blueberry)		
BLUEBERRY PRESERVE OR JAM:		
Sweetened (Smucker's)	1 T.	53
Dietetic (Dia-Mel)	1 T.	6
BLUEFISH, broiled	3½″ × 3″ × ½″ piece	199
BODY BUDDIES, cereal (General Mills):		
Brown sugar & honey	1 cup	110
Natural fruit flavor	¾ cup	110
BOLOGNA:		
(Best's Kosher):		
Chub	1-oz. serving	90
Sliced	1-oz. serving	68
(Eckrich):		
Beef, garlic, pickled, ring or sliced	1 oz.	95
Thick sliced	1.7-oz. slice	160
(Hormel):		
Beef	1-oz. slice	86
Fine ground, ring	1-oz. serving	82
Meat	1-oz. slice	85
(Oscar Mayer):		
Beef	.8-oz. slice	73
Beef	1-oz. slice	90
Beef	1.3-oz. slice	120
Meat	.8-oz. slice	74
Meat	1-oz. slice	91
(Swift)	1-oz. slice	95
(Vienna) beef	1-oz. serving	84
BOLOGNA & CHEESE		
(Oscar Mayer)	.8-oz. slice	73

Food and Description	Measure or Quantity	Calories
BONITO, canned (Star-Kist):		
Chunk	6½-oz. can	604
Solid	7-oz. can	650
BOO*BERRY, cereal (General Mills)	1 cup	110
BORSCHT, canned:		
Regular:		
(Gold's)	8-oz. serving	72
(Mother's) old fashioned	8-oz. serving	90
Dietetic or low calorie:		
(Gold's)	8-oz. serving	24
(Mother's):		
Artificially sweetened	8-oz. serving	29
Unsalted	8-oz. serving	107
(Rokeach)	8-oz. serving	27
BOSCO (See SYRUP)		
*BOWL O'NOODLES (Nestlé), beef or chicken	1½-oz. envelope	160
BOYSENBERRY JELLY:		
Sweetened (Smucker's)	1 T.	53
Dietetic		
BOYSENBERRY SPREAD, low sugar:		
(Smucker's)	1 T.	24
(S&W) *Nutradiet*	1 T.	12
BRAN, crude	1 oz.	60
BRAN, Miller's	1 oz.	87
BRAN BREAKFAST CEREAL:		
(Crawford's) & dates	⅓ cup	100
(Kellogg's):		
All Bran or *Bran Buds*	⅓ cup	70
Cracklin' Bran	½ cup	110
40% bran flakes	¾ cup	90
Raisin	¾ cup	110
(Nabisco)	½ cup	70
(Post) 40% bran flakes	⅔ cup	107
(Quaker) *Corn Bran*	⅔ cup	109
(Ralston-Purina):		
Bran Chex	⅔ cup	90
40% bran	¾ cup	100
Raisin	¾ cup	120
BRANDY, FLAVORED (Mr. Boston):		
Apricot	1 fl. oz.	94
Blackberry	1 fl. oz.	92
Cherry	1 fl. oz.	87
Coffee	1 fl. oz.	100
Ginger	1 fl. oz.	72
Peach	1 fl. oz.	94

15

Food and Description	Measure or Quantity	Calories
BRAUNSCHWEIGER:		
(Oscar Mayer) chub	1 oz.	98
(Swift) 8-oz. chub	1 oz.	109
BRAZIL NUT:		
Shelled	4 nuts	114
Roasted (Fisher) salted	1-oz. serving	193
BREAD:		
Apple (Pepperidge Farm) with cinnamon	.9-oz. slice	70
Boston Brown	3″ × ¾″ slice	101
Cinnamon (Pepperidge Farm)	.9-oz. slice	80
Corn & Molasses (Pepperidge Farm)	.9-oz. slice	75
Cracked wheat (Pepperidge Farm)	1 slice	75
Crispbread, *Wasa*:		
Mora	3.2-oz. slice	333
Rye, golden	.4-oz. slice	37
Rye, lite	.3-oz. slice	30
Sesame	.5-oz. slice	50
Sport	.4-oz. slice	42
Date nut roll (Dromedary)	1-oz. slice	80
Date walnut (Pepperidge Farm)	.9-oz. slice	75
Flatbread, *Ideal:*		
Bran	.2-oz. slice	19
Extra thin	.1-oz. slice	12
Whole grain	.2-oz. slice	19
French:		
(Pepperidge Farm)	2-oz. slice	150
(Wonder)	1-oz. slice	75
Hillbilly	1-oz. slice	72
Hollywood, dark	1-oz. slice	72
Honey bran (Pepperidge Farm)	1 slice	95
Honey, wheat berry (Arnold)	1.2-oz. slice	90
Italian (Pepperidge Farm)	2-oz. slice	150
Low sodium (Wonder)	1-oz. slice	71
Oatmeal (Pepperidge Farm)	.9-oz. slice	70
Orange & Raisin (Pepperidge Farm)	.9-oz. slice	70
Protogen Protein (Thomas')	.7-oz. slice	46
Pumpernickel:		
(Arnold)	1-oz. slice	75
(Levy's)	1.1-oz. slice	85
(Pepperidge Farm):		
Regular	1.1-oz. slice	85
Party	.2-oz. slice	17
Raisin:		
(Arnold) tea	.9-oz. slice	70
(Pepperidge Farm)	1 slice	75
(Sun-Maid)	1-oz. slice	80
(Thomas') cinnamon	.8-oz. slice	60

Food and Description	Measure or Quantity	Calories
Roman Meal	1-oz. slice	77
Rye:		
(Arnold) Jewish	1.1-oz. slice	75
(Levy's) real	1-oz. slice	80
(Pepperidge Farm) family	1.1-oz. slice	85
(Wonder)	1-oz. slice	69
Sahara (Thomas')	1-oz. piece	85
Sour dough, *Di Carlo*	1-oz. slice	70
Sprouted wheat (Pepperidge Farm)	.9-oz. slice	113
Vienna (Pepperidge Farm)	.9-oz. slice	175
Wheat:		
(Arnold) *Bran'nola*	1.3-oz. slice	105
Fresh Horizons	1-oz. slice	54
Fresh & Natural	1-oz. slice	77
Home Pride	1-oz. slice	73
(Pepperidge Farm) sandwich	.8-oz. slice	55
(Wonder) family	1-oz. slice	75
Wheatberry, *Home Pride,* honey	1-oz. slice	74
Wheat Germ (Pepperidge Farm)	.9-oz. slice	70
White:		
(Arnold):		
Brick Oven	.8-oz. slice	65
Measure Up	.5-oz. slice	40
Melba Thin	.5-oz. slice	40
Home Pride	1-oz. slice	72
(Pepperidge Farm):		
Large loaf	.9-oz. slice	75
Sandwich	.8-oz. slice	65
Sliced, 1-lb. loaf	.9-oz. slice	75
Toasting	1.2-oz. slice	85
(Wonder) regular	1-oz. slice	70
Whole wheat:		
(Arnold) *Brick Oven*	.8-oz. slice	60
(Arnold) *Measure Up*	.5-oz. slice	40
(Pepperidge Farm) thin slice	1 slice	70
(Thomas') 100%	.8-oz. slice	56
BREAD, CANNED, brown, plain or raisin (B&M)	½" slice	80
BREAD CRUMBS (Contadina) seasoned	½ cup	211
***BREAD DOUGH,** frozen:		
(Pepperidge Farm):		
Country rye or white	⅒ of loaf	80
Stone ground wheat	⅒ of loaf	75
(Rich's):		
French	¹⁄₂₀ of loaf	59
Italian	¹⁄₂₀ of loaf	60
Wheat	.5-oz. slice	60

Food and Description	Measure or Quantity	Calories
White	.8-oz. slice	56
*BREAD MIX (Pillsbury):		
Applesauce spice, banana or blueberry nut	½₁₂ of loaf	150
Cherry nut or nut	½₁₂ of loaf	170
Cranberry or date	½₁₂ of loaf	160
BREAD PUDDING, with raisins	½ cup	248
BREAKFAST BAR (Carnation):		
Almond crunch	1 piece	210
All other varieties	1 piece	200
*BREAKFAST DRINK (Pillsbury)	1 pouch	290
BREAKFAST SQUARES (General Mills) all flavors	1 bar	190
BRIGHT & EARLY	6 fl. oz.	90
BROCCOLI:		
Boiled, whole stalk	1 stalk	47
Boiled, ½" pieces	½ cup	20
Frozen:		
(Birds Eye) in cheese sauce	⅓ pkg.	112
(Birds Eye) in Hollandaise sauce	⅓ pkg.	105
(Green Giant) spears in butter sauce	⅓ pkg.	40
(Green Giant):		
Cuts, polybag	½ cup	18
Harvest Fresh	4 oz.	33
Spears in butter sauce	3⅓ oz.	40
(McKenzie) chopped or spears	⅓ pkg.	25
(Mrs. Paul's) in cheese sauce	⅓ pkg.	162
(Seabrook Farms) chopped or spears	⅓ pkg.	30
BROTH & SEASONING:		
(George Washington)	1 packet	5
Maggi	1 T.	22
BRUSSELS SPROUT:		
Boiled	3–4 sprouts	28
Frozen:		
(Birds Eye) baby with cheese sauce	⅓ pkg.	104
(Birds Eye) baby, deluxe	⅓ pkg.	49
(Green Giant) in butter sauce	⅓ pkg.	50
(Green Giant) halves in cheese sauce	⅓ pkg.	64
(Stouffer's) au gratin	⅓ pkg.	124
BUCKWHEAT, cracked (Pocono)	1 oz.	104
BUC*WHEATS, cereal (General Mills)	1 oz. (¾ cup)	110
BULGUR, canned, seasoned	4 oz. serving	206
BULLWINKLE PUDDING STIX, *Good Humor*	2 ½-fl. oz. bar	120

18

Food and Description	Measure or Quantity	Calories
BURGER KING:		
Apple pie	3-oz. pie	240
Cheeseburger	1 burger	350
Cheeseburger, double meat	1 burger	530
Coca Cola	1 medium-sized drink	121
French fries	1 regular order	210
Hamburger	1 burger	290
Onion rings	1 regular order	270
Pepsi, diet	1 medium-sized drink	7
Shake, chocolate or vanilla	1 shake	340
Whopper:		
Regular	1 burger	630
Regular, with cheese	1 burger	740
Double beef	1 burger	850
Double beef, with cheese	1 burger	950
Junior	1 burger	370
Junior, with cheese	1 burger	420
BURGUNDY WINE:		
(Italian Swiss Colony)	3 fl. oz.	61
(Louis M. Martini)	3 fl. oz.	90
(Paul Masson)	3 fl. oz.	70
(Taylor)	3 fl. oz.	75
BURGUNDY WINE, SPARKLING:		
(B&G)	3 fl. oz.	69
(Great Western)	3 fl. oz.	82
(Taylor)	3 fl. oz.	78
BURRITO:		
*Canned (Del Monte)	1 burrito	310
Frozen:		
(Hormel):		
Beef	1 burrito	220
Cheese	1 burrito	250
Hot chili	1 burrito	210
(Van de Kamp's) & guacamole sauce	½ of 12-oz. pkg.	350
BURRITO FILLING MIX, canned (Del Monte)	1 cup	220
BUTTER:		
Regular (Breakstone)	1 T.	100
Regular (Meadow Gold)	1 tsp.	35
Whipped (Breakstone)	1 T.	67
BUTTERSCOTCH MORSELS (Nestlé)	1 oz.	150

C

CABBAGE:
  Canned:
    (Comstock) red, solids & liq. — ½ cup — 60
    (Greenwood's) red, solids & liq. — ½ cup — 60
  Frozen (Green Giant) stuffed — 7-oz. serving — 174
CABERNET SAUVIGNON
  (Paul Masson) — 1 fl. oz. — 70
CAFE COMFORT, 55 proof — 1 fl. oz. — 79
CAKE:
  Regular, non-frozen:
    Plain, home recipe, with butter,
      with boiled white icing — ⅑ of 9″ square — 401
    Angel food, home recipe — 1/12 of 8″ cake — 108
    Caramel, home recipe, with
      caramel icing — ⅑ of 9″ square — 322
    Carrot (Hostess) — 3-oz. piece — 319
    Chocolate, home recipe, with
      chocolate icing, 2-layer — 1/12 of 9″ cake — 365
    Crumb (Hostess) — 1¼-oz. cake — 131
    Fruit:
      Home recipe, dark — 1/30 of 8″ loaf — 57
      Home recipe, light, made with
        butter — 1/30 of 8″ loaf — 58
      (Holland Honey Cake) unsalted — 1/14 of cake — 80
    Pound, home recipe, traditional,
      made with butter — 3½″ × 3½″ slice — 123
    Raisin Date Loaf (Holland Honey
      Cake) low sodium — 1/14 of 13-oz. cake — 80
    Sponge, home recipe — 1/12 of 10″ cake — 196
    White, home recipe, made with
      butter, without icing, 2-layer — ⅑ of 9″ wide, 3″ high cake — 353
    Yellow, home recipe, made with
      butter, without icing, 2-layer — 1/19 of cake — 351
  Frozen:
    Apple Walnut:
      (Pepperidge Farm) with cream
        cheese icing — ⅛ of 11¾-oz. cake — 150
      (Sara Lee) — ⅛ of 12½-oz. cake — 165
    Banana (Sara Lee) — ⅛ of 13¾-oz. cake — 175
    Black forest (Sara Lee) — ⅛ of 21-oz. cake — 203
    Boston Cream (Pepperidge Farm) — ¼ of 11¾-oz. cake — 290

Food and Description	Measure or Quantity	Calories
Carrot (Sara Lee)	⅛ of 12¼-oz. cake	152
Cheesecake:		
(Morton) *Great Little Desserts:*		
Cherry	6½-oz. cake	476
Cream	6½-oz. cake	489
Strawberry	6½-oz. cake	491
(Rich's) Viennese	1/14 of 42-oz. cake	230
(Sara Lee):		
Blueberry, *For 2*	½ of 11.3-oz. cake	425
Cream cheese	⅓ of 10-oz. cake	281
Cream cheese, blueberry	⅙ of 19-oz. cake	233
Cream cheese, cherry	⅙ of 19-oz. cake	225
Cream cheese, strawberry	⅙ of 19-oz. cake	223
Cream cheese, strawberry, French	⅛ of 26-oz. cake	258
Strawberry, *For 2*	½ of 11.3-oz. cake	420
Chocolate:		
(Pepperidge Farm):		
Layer, fudge	1/10 of 17-oz. cake	190
Rich 'N Moist with chocolate icing	⅛ of 14¼-oz. cake	190
Supreme	¼ of 11½-oz. cake	310
(Sara Lee):		
Regular	⅛ of 13¼-oz. cake	199
German	⅛ of 12¼-oz. cake	173
Layer 'N Cream	⅛ of 18-oz. cake	215
Coffee (Sara Lee):		
Almond	⅛ of 11¾-oz. cake	165
Almond ring	⅛ of 9½-oz. cake	135
Apple	⅛ of 15-oz. cake	175
Apple, *For 2*	½ of 9-oz. cake	419
Butter, *For 2*	½ of 6½-oz. cake	356
Maple crunch ring	⅛ of 9¾-oz. cake	138
Pecan	⅛ of 11¼-oz. cake	163
Streusel, butter	⅛ of 11½-oz. cake	164
Streusel, cinnamon	⅛ of 10.9-oz. cake	154
Crumb (see ROLL OR BUN, Crumb)		
Devil's food (Pepperidge Farm) layer	1/10 of 17-oz. cake	180
Golden (Pepperidge Farm) layer	1/10 of 17-oz. cake	180
Lemon coconut (Pepperidge Farm)	¼ of 12¼-oz. cake	280
Orange (Sara Lee)	⅛ of 13¾-oz. cake	179
Pineapple cream (Pepperidge Farm) Supreme	1/12 24-oz. cake	180
Pound (Sara Lee):		
Regular	1/10 of 10¾-oz. cake	125
Banana nut	1/10 of 11-oz. cake	117

Food and Description	Measure or Quantity	Calories
Chocolate	1/10 of 10¾-oz. cake	122
Family size	1/15 of 16½-oz. cake	127
Homestyle	1/10 of 9½-oz. cake	114
Strawberry cream (Pepperidge Farm) Supreme	1/12 of 12-oz. cake	190
Strawberries 'n cream, layer (Sara Lee)	1/8 of 20½-oz. cake	218
Torte (Sara Lee):		
Apples 'n cream	1/8 of 21-oz. cake	203
Fudge & nut	1/8 of 15¾-oz. cake	200
Vanilla (Pepperidge Farm) layer	1/10 of 17-oz. cake	180
Walnut, layer (Sara Lee)	1/8 of 18-oz. cake	210
CAKE OR COOKIE ICING		
(Pillsbury) all flavors	1 T.	70
CAKE ICING:		
Butter pecan (Betty Crocker) *Creamy Deluxe*	1/12 of can	170
Caramel, home recipe	4 oz.	408
Cherry (Betty Crocker) *Creamy Deluxe*	1/12 of can	170
Chocolate:		
(Betty Crocker) *Creamy Deluxe:*		
Regular	1/12 of can	170
Chip	1/12 of can	170
Milk	1/12 of can	170
Sour cream	1/12 of can	160
(Duncan Hines)	1/12 of can	163
(Pillsbury) *Frosting Supreme:*		
Fudge	1/12 of can	160
Milk	1/12 of can	160
Coconut almond (Pillsbury) *Frosting Supreme*	1/12 of can	150
Cream cheese:		
(Betty Crocker) *Creamy Deluxe*	1/12 of can	170
(Pillsbury) *Frosting Supreme*	1/12 of can	160
Double dutch (Pillsbury) *Frosting Supreme*	1/12 of can	160
Orange (Betty Crocker) *Creamy Deluxe*	1/12 of can	170
Strawberry (Pillsbury) *Frosting Supreme*	1/12 of can	160
Vanilla:		
(Betty Crocker) *Creamy Deluxe*	1/12 of can	170
(Duncan Hines)	1/12 of can	163
(Pillsbury) *Frosting Supreme*	1/12 of can	160
White:		
Home recipe, boiled	4 oz.	358
Home recipe, uncooked	4 oz.	426

Food and Description	Measure or Quantity	Calories
(Betty Crocker) *Creamy Deluxe*	¹⁄₁₂ of can	160
*CAKE ICING MIX:		
Regular:		
Banana (Betty Crocker) *Chiquita*, creamy	¹⁄₁₂ of pkg.	170
Butter Brickle (Betty Crocker) creamy	¹⁄₁₂ of pkg.	170
Butter pecan (Betty Crocker) creamy	¹⁄₁₂ of pkg.	170
Caramel (Pillsbury) *Rich'n Easy*	¹⁄₁₂ of pkg.	140
Cherry (Betty Crocker) creamy	¹⁄₁₂ of pkg.	170
Chocolate:		
Home recipe, fudge	½ cup	586
(Betty Crocker) creamy:		
Fluffy, almond fudge	¹⁄₁₂ of pkg.	180
Fudge, creamy, dark or milk	¹⁄₁₂ of pkg.	170
(Pillsbury) *Rich 'N Easy*, fudge or milk	¹⁄₁₂ of pkg.	150
Coconut almond (Pillsbury)	¹⁄₁₂ of pkg.	160
Coconut pecan:		
(Betty Crocker) creamy	¹⁄₁₂ of pkg.	140
(Pillsbury)	¹⁄₁₂ of pkg.	150
Cream cheese & nut (Betty Crocker) creamy	¹⁄₁₂ of pkg.	150
Lemon:		
(Betty Crocker) *Sunkist*, creamy	¹⁄₁₂ of pkg.	170
(Pillsbury) *Rich 'N Easy*	¹⁄₁₂ of pkg.	140
Strawberry (Pillsbury) *Rich 'N Easy*	¹⁄₁₂ of pkg.	140
Vanilla (Pillsbury) *Rich 'N Easy*	¹⁄₁₂ of pkg.	150
White:		
(Betty Crocker) fluffy	¹⁄₁₂ of pkg.	60
(Betty Crocker) sour cream, creamy	¹⁄₁₂ of pkg.	180
(Pillsbury) fluffy	¹⁄₁₂ of pkg.	60
Dietetic (Betty Crocker) *Lite* chocolate, lemon or vanilla	¹⁄₁₂ of pkg.	100
CAKE MIX:		
Regular:		
Angel Food:		
(Betty Crocker):		
Chocolate or one-step	¹⁄₁₂ pkg.	140
Traditional	¹⁄₁₂ pkg.	130
(Duncan Hines)	¹⁄₁₂ pkg.	124
*(Pillsbury) raspberry or white	¹⁄₁₂ of cake	140
Applesauce raisin (Betty Crocker) *Snackin' Cake*	¹⁄₉ pkg.	180

Food and Description	Measure or Quantity	Calories
*Applesauce spice (Pillsbury) *Pillsbury Plus*	1/12 of cake	250
Banana:		
*(Betty Crocker) *Supermoist*	1/12 of cake	260
*(Pillsbury) *Pillsbury Plus*	1/12 of cake	260
Banana walnut (Betty Crocker) *Snackin' Cake*	1/9 pkg.	190
*Boston cream (Pillsbury) *Bundt*	1/16 of cake	270
*Butter (Pillsbury):		
Pillsbury Plus	1/12 of cake	240
Streusel Swirl, rich	1/16 of cake	260
Butter Brickle (Betty Crocker) *Supermoist*	1/12 of cake	260
*Butter pecan (Betty Crocker) *Supermoist*	1/12 of cake	250
*Carrot (Betty Crocker) *Supermoist*	1/12 of cake	260
*Carrot 'n spice (Pillsbury) *Pillsbury Plus*	1/12 of cake	260
*Cheesecake:		
(Jell-O)	1/8 of 8" cake	250
(Royal)	1/8 of cake	230
*Cherry chip (Betty Crocker) *Supermoist*	1/12 of cake	180
Chocolate:		
(Betty Crocker):		
*Pudding	1/6 of cake	230
Snackin' Cake:		
Almond	1/9 pkg.	200
Fudge chip	1/9 pkg.	190
Stir 'N Frost:		
with chocolate frosting	1/6 pkg.	220
Fudge, with vanilla frosting	1/6 pkg.	220
Supermoist:		
*Fudge	1/12 of cake	250
*Milk	1/12 of cake	250
*Sour cream	1/12 of cake	260
*(Pillsbury):		
Bundt:		
Fudge nut crown	1/16 of cake	220
Fudge, tunnel of	1/16 of cake	270
Macaroon	1/16 of cake	250
Pillsbury Plus:		
Fudge, dark	1/12 of cake	260
Fudge, marble	1/12 of cake	270
Mint	1/12 of cake	260
Streusel Swirl, German	1/16 of cake	260

Food and Description	Measure or Quantity	Calories
*Cinnamon (Pillsbury) *Streusel Swirl*	1/16 of cake	260
Coconut pecan (Betty Crocker) *Snackin' Cake*	1/9 of pkg.	190
Coffee cake:		
*(Aunt Jemima)	1/8 of cake	170
*(Pillsbury):		
Apple cinnamon	1/8 of cake	240
Cinnamon streusel	1/8 of cake	250
Date nut (Betty Crocker) *Snackin' Cake*	1/9 of pkg.	190
Devil's food:		
*(Betty Crocker) *Supermoist*	1/12 of cake	260
(Duncan Hines) deluxe	1/12 of pkg.	190
*(Pillsbury) *Pillsbury Plus*	1/12 of cake	250
Fudge (See Chocolate)		
Golden chocolate chip (Betty Crocker) *Snackin' Cake*	1/9 of pkg.	190
Lemon:		
(Betty Crocker):		
*Chiffon	1/12 of cake	190
Stir 'N Frost, with lemon frosting	1/12 of pkg.	230
Supermoist	1/12 of cake	260
*(Pillsbury):		
Bundt, tunnel of	1/16 of cake	270
Streusel Swirl	1/16 of cake	260
*Lemon blueberry (Pillsbury) *Bundt*	1/16 of cake	200
Marble:		
*(Betty Crocker) *Supermoist*	1/12 of cake	260
*(Pillsbury):		
Bundt, supreme, ring	1/16 of cake	250
Streusel Swirl, fudge	1/16 of cake	260
*Oats 'n brown sugar (Pillsbury) *Pillsbury Plus*	1/12 of cake	230
*Orange (Betty Crocker) *Supermoist*	1/12 of cake	260
Pound:		
*(Betty Crocker) golden	1/12 of cake	200
*(Dromedary)	3/4" slice	210
*(Pillsbury) *Bundt*	1/16 of cake	230
Spice (Betty Crocker):		
Snackin' Cake, raisin	1/9 of pkg.	180
Stir N' Frost, with vanilla frosting	1/6 of cake	270
Supermoist	1/12 of cake	260

Food and Description	Measure or Quantity	Calories
Strawberry:		
*(Betty Crocker) *Supermoist*	¹⁄₁₂ of cake	260
*(Pillsbury) *Pillsbury Plus*	¹⁄₁₂ of cake	260
*Upside down (Betty Crocker) pineapple	¹⁄₉ of cake	270
White:		
*(Betty Crocker):		
Stir 'N Frost, with chocolate frosting	¹⁄₆ of cake	220
Supermoist	¹⁄₁₂ of cake	230
(Duncan Hines) deluxe	¹⁄₁₂ of pkg.	188
*(Pillsbury) *Pillsbury Plus*	¹⁄₁₂ of cake	240
Yellow:		
*(Betty Crocker) *Supermoist*	¹⁄₁₂ of cake	260
(Duncan Hines) deluxe	¹⁄₁₂ of pkg.	188
*(Pillsbury) *Pillsbury Plus*	¹⁄₁₂ of cake	260
*(Swans Down)	¹⁄₁₂ of cake	185
*Dietetic (Estee):		
Chocolate	¹⁄₁₀ of cake	100
Lemon	¹⁄₁₀ of cake	91
White	¹⁄₁₀ of cake	85
CAMPARI, 45 proof	1 fl. oz.	66
CANDY, REGULAR:		
Almond, chocolate covered (Hershey's) *Golden Almond*	1 oz.	163
Almond Cluster (Heath)	1 oz.	142
Almond, Jordan (Banner)	1¼-oz. box	154
Apricot Delight (Sahadi)	1 oz.	100
Baby Ruth	1.8-oz. piece	260
Bridge Mix (Nabisco)	1 piece	8
Bun Bars (Wayne)	1 oz.	133
Butter Brickle Bar (Heath)	1 oz.	150
Butterfinger	1.6-oz. bar	220
Butterscotch Skimmers (Nabisco)	1 piece	25
Caramel:		
Caramel Flipper (Wayne)	1 oz.	128
Caramel Nip (Pearson)	1 piece	29
Caramel Pattie (Heath)	1-oz. serving	113
Cereal Raisin Bar (Heath)	2-oz. serving	296
Charleston Chew	1½-oz. bar	179
Cherry, chocolate-covered (Nabisco; *Welch's*)	1 piece	66
Chocolate bar:		
Choco-Lite (Nestlé)	.27-oz. bar	41
Choco-Lite (Nestlé)	1-oz. serving	150
Crunch (Nestlé)	1¹⁄₁₆-oz. bar	159
Krunch (Heath)	1½-oz. serving	221

Food and Description	Measure or Quantity	Calories
Milk:		
(Heath) crunch with toffee	2¼-oz. serving	334
(Heath) solid	2¼-oz. serving	339
(Hershey's)	1.2-oz. bar	187
(Hershey's)	4-oz. bar	623
(Nestlé)	.35-oz. bar	53
(Nestlé)	1¹⁄₁₆-oz. bar	159
Special Dark (Hershey's)	1.05-oz. bar	160
Special Dark (Hershey's)	4-oz. bar	611
Chocolate bar with almonds:		
(Heath)	2½-oz. serving	388
(Hershey's) milk	.35-oz. bar	55
(Hershey's) milk	1.15-oz. bar	180
(Hershey's) milk	4-oz. bar	625
(Nestlé)	1-oz. serving	150
Chocolate Parfait (Pearson)	1 piece	31
Chuckles	1 oz.	93
Clark Bar	1.4-oz. bar	188
Clark Bar	1.65-oz. bar	222
Cluster, peanut, chocolate-covered (Hoffman)	1 cluster	205
Coffee Nip (Pearson)	1 piece	29
Coffioca (Pearson)	1 piece	31
Crispy Bar (Clark)	1¼-oz. bar	187
Crows (Mason)	1 piece	11
Dots (Mason)	1 piece	11
Dutch Treat Bar (Clark)	1¹⁄₁₆-oz. bar	160
Fudge (Nabisco) bar, *Home Style*	1 bar	90
Good & Plenty	1 oz.	100
Halvah (Sahadi) original & marble	1 oz.	150
Hollywood	1½-oz. bar	185
Jelly bean (Curtiss)	1 piece	12
Jelly rings, *Chuckles*	1 piece	37
Jujubes, *Chuckles*	1 piece	13
Ju Jus:		
Assorted	1 piece	7
Coins or raspberries	1 piece	15
Kisses (Hershey's)	1 piece	27
Kit Kat	.6-oz. bar	80
Krackel Bar	.35-oz. bar	52
Krackel Bar	1.2-oz. bar	178
Licorice:		
Licorice Nips (Pearson)	1 piece	29
(Switzer) bars, bites or stix:		
Black	1 oz.	94
Cherry or strawberry	1 oz.	98
Chocolate	1 oz.	97

Food and Description	Measure or Quantity	Calories
Twist:		
Black (American Licorice Co.)	1 piece	27
Black (Curtiss)	1 piece	27
Red (American Licorice Co.)	1 piece	33
Life Savers, drop	1 piece	10
Life Savers, mint	1 piece	7
Lollipops (Life Savers)	.9-oz. pop	99
Mallo Cup (Boyer)	9/16-oz. piece	54
Malted milk balls (Brach's)	1 piece	9
Mars Bar (M&M/Mars)	1½-oz. serving	203
Marshmallow (Campfire)	1 oz.	111
Mary Jane (Miller):		
Small size	¼ oz.	19
Large size	1½-oz. bar	110
Milk Duds (Clark)	¾-oz. box	89
Milk Duds (Clark)	1¼-oz. box	148
Milky Way (M&M/Mars)	.8-oz. bar	100
Milky Way (M&M/Mars)	1.9-oz. serving	238
Mint or peppermint:		
After dinner (Richardson):		
Jelly center	1 oz.	104
Regular	1 oz.	109
Chocolate-covered (Richardson)	1 oz.	106
Jamaica or *Liberty Mints* (Nabisco)	1 piece	24
Meltaway (Heath)	1 oz.	156
Mint Parfait (Pearson)	1 piece	31
Junior mint pattie (Nabisco)	1 piece	10
Peppermint pattie (Nabisco)	1 piece	64
M & M's:		
Peanut	1½ oz.	217
Plain	1½-oz.	210
Mr. Goodbar (Hershey's)	.35-oz. bar	54
Mr. Goodbar (Hershey's)	1½-oz. bar	233
$100,000 Bar (Nestlé)	1¼-oz. bar	175
Orange slices (Curtiss)	1 piece	29
Peanut, chocolate-covered:		
(Curtiss)	1 piece	5
(Nabisco)	1 piece	24
Peanut crunch (Sahadi)	¾-oz. bar	110
Peanut, French burnt (Curtiss)	1 piece	4
Peanut brittle (Planters):		
Jumbo Peanut Block Bar	1 oz.	119
Jumbo Peanut Block Bar	1 piece (4 grams)	61
Peanut butter cup:		
(Boyer)	1.5-oz. pkg.	148
(Reese's)	.6-oz. cup	92

Food and Description	Measure or Quantity	Calories
Raisin, chocolate-covered:		
(Nabisco)	1 piece	4
Raisinets (BB)	5¢ size	140
Reggie Bar	2-oz. bar	290
Rolo (Hershey's)	1 piece	30
Royals, mint chocolate (M&M/Mars)	1½-oz. serving	209
Sesame crunch (Sahadi)	¾-oz. bar	110
Snickers	1.8-oz. bar	249
Spearmint leaves:		
(Curtiss)	1 piece	32
(Nabisco) *Chuckles*	1 piece	27
Starburst (M&M/Mars)	1-oz. serving	118
Sugar Babies (Nabisco)	1 piece	6
Sugar Daddy (Nabisco):		
Caramel sucker	1 piece	121
Nugget	1 piece	27
Sugar Mama (Nabisco)	1 piece	101
Summit, cookie bar (M&M/Mars)	1-oz. serving	144
Taffy:		
Salt water (Brach's)	1 piece	31
Turkish (Bonomo)	1-oz. bar	108
3 Musketeers	.8-oz. bar	99
3 Musketeers	2-oz. serving	255
Toffee Brickle (Heath)	1 oz.	156
Tootsie Roll:		
Chocolate	.23-oz. midgee	26
Chocolate	¹⁄₁₆-oz. bar	72
Chocolate	¾-oz. bar	86
Chocolate	1-oz. bar	115
Chocolate	1¾-oz. bar	201
Flavored	.6-oz. square	19
Pop, all flavors	.49-oz. pop	55
Pop drop, all flavors	4.7-gram piece	19
Twix, cookie bar (M&M/Mars)	1¾-oz. serving	246
Twix, peanut butter cookie bar (M&M/Mars)	1¾-oz. serving	261
Twizzlers:		
Cherry, chocolate or strawberry	1 oz.	100
Licorice	1 oz.	90
Whatchamacallit (Hershey's)	1.15-oz. bar	176
World Series Bar	1 oz.	128
Zagnut Bar (Clark)	.7-oz. bar	92
CANDY, DIETETIC:		
Carob bar, *Joan's Natural:*		
Coconut	1 section of 3-oz. bar	43
Coconut	3-oz. bar	516

Food and Description	Measure or Quantity	Calories
Fruit & nut	1 section of 3-oz. bar	46
Fruit & nut	3-oz. bar	559
Honey bran	1 section of 3-oz. bar	40
Honey bran	3-oz. bar	487
Peanut	1 section of 3-oz. bar	43
Peanut	3-oz. bar	521
Chocolate or chocolate flavored bar (Estee):		
Bittersweet	1 section of 2½-oz. bar	35
Bittersweet	2½-oz. bar	417
Coconut	1 section of 2½-oz. bar	35
Coconut	2½-oz. bar	420
Crunch	1 section of 2-oz. bar	34
Crunch	2-oz. bar	407
Fruit & nut	1 section of 2½-oz. bar	33
Fruit & nut	2½-oz. bar	398
Milk	1 section of 2½-oz. bar	34
Milk	2½-oz. bar	413
Toasted bran	1 section of 2½-oz. bar	33
Toasted bran	2½-oz. bar	398
Chocolate bar with almonds (Estee) milk	1 section of 2½-oz. bar	35
Chocolate bar with almonds (Estee) milk	2½-oz. bar	415
Estee-ets, with peanuts (Estee)	1 piece	7
Gum drops (Estee) any flavor	1 piece	3
Hard candy:		
(Estee) assorted fruit or peppermint	1 piece	11
(Estee) Tropi-mix	1 piece	10
Mint:		
(Estee) *Esteemints*, all flavors	1 piece	4
(Sunkist):		
Mini mint	1 piece	<1
Roll mint	1 piece	4
Peanut butter cup (Estee)	1 cup	50
Raisins, chocolate-covered (Estee)	1 piece	6
CANNELLONI FLORENTINE, frozen (Weight Watchers) one-compartment	13-oz. meal	450

Food and Description	Measure or Quantity	Calories
CANTALOUPE, cubed	½ cup	24
CAPERS (Crosse & Blackwell)	1 tsp.	2
CAP'N CRUNCH, cereal (Quaker):		
Regular	¾ cup	121
Crunchberry	¾ cup	120
Peanut butter	¾ cup	127
CARAWAY SEED (French's)	1 tsp.	8
CARNATION INSTANT BREAKFAST:		
Bar:		
Chocolate chip	1 bar	200
Peanut butter crunch	1 bar	180
Packets, all flavors	1 packet	130
CARROT:		
Raw	5½" × 1" carrot	21
Boiled, slices	½ cup	24
Canned, regular:		
(Del Monte) drained	½ cup	30
(Libby's) solids & liq.	½ cup	20
(Stokely-Van Camp) solids & liq.	½ cup	25
Canned, dietetic:		
(Featherweight) solids & liq.	½ cup	30
(S&W) *Nutradiet,* sliced, solids & liq.	½ cup	30
Frozen:		
(Birds Eye) with brown sugar glaze	⅓ pkg.	84
(Green Giant) cuts in butter sauce	⅓ pkg.	76
(McKenzie)	⅓ pkg.	40
(Seabrook Farms)	⅓ pkg.	39
CASABA MELON	1-lb. melon	61
CASHEW NUT:		
(Fisher):		
Dry roasted	1 oz.	156
Oil roasted	1 oz.	159
(Planters):		
Dry roasted	1 oz.	160
Oil roasted	1 oz.	170
CATSUP:		
Regular:		
(Del Monte)	1 T.	17
(Smucker's)	1 T.	21
Dietetic:		
(Featherweight)	1 T.	6
(Tillie Lewis) *Tasti Diet*	1 T.	8
CAULIFLOWER:		
Raw or boiled buds	½ cup	14
Frozen:		
(Birds Eye) florets, deluxe	⅓ pkg.	28

31

Food and Description	Measure or Quantity	Calories
(Green Giant) in cheese sauce	3⅓ oz.	53
(Mrs. Paul's) light batter & cheese	⅓ pkg.	135
(Seabrook Farms)	⅓ pkg.	23
(Stouffer's) au gratin	5-oz. serving	157
CAVIAR:		
Pressed	1 oz.	90
Whole eggs	1 T.	42
CELERY:		
1 large outer stalk	8″ × 1½″ at root end	7
Diced or cut	½ cup	9
Salt (French's)	1 tsp.	2
Seed (French's)	1 tsp.	11
CERTS	1 piece	6
CHABLIS WINE:		
(Almaden) light	3 fl. oz.	42
(Gallo)	3 fl. oz.	61
(Great Western)	3 fl. oz.	70
(Paul Masson) regular	3 fl. oz.	71
(Paul Masson) light	3 fl. oz.	45
CHAMPAGNE:		
(Bollinger)	3 fl. oz.	72
(Great Western):		
Regular	3 fl. oz.	71
Brut	3 fl. oz.	74
Pink	3 fl. oz.	81
(Taylor) dry	3 fl. oz.	78
CHARLOTTE RUSSE, homemade recipe	4 oz.	324
CHEERIOS, cereal, regular or honey & nut	1 oz.	110
CHEESE:		
American or cheddar:		
Cube, natural	1″ cube	68
(Featherweight) low sodium	1 oz.	110
Laughing Cow	1 oz.	110
(Sargento):		
Midget, regular or sharp	1 oz.	114
Shredded, non-dairy	1 oz.	90
Wispride, sharp	1 oz.	115
Blue:		
(Frigo)	1 oz.	100
Laughing Cow:		
Cube	⅙ oz.	12
Wedge	¾ oz.	55
(Sargento): cold pack or crumbled	1 oz.	100
Brick (Sargento)	1 oz.	105
Brie (Sargento) *Danish Danko*	1 oz.	80

Food and Description	Measure or Quantity	Calories
Burgercheese (Sargento) *Danish Danko*	1 oz.	106
Camembert (Sargento) *Danish Danko*	1 oz.	88
Colby:		
(Featherweight) low sodium	1 oz.	100
(Pauly) low sodium	1 oz.	115
(Sargento) shredded or sliced	1 oz.	112
Cottage:		
Unflavored:		
(Bison):		
Regular	1 oz.	29
Dietetic	1 oz.	22
(Dairylea)	1 oz.	30
(Friendship)	1 oz.	30
Flavored (Friendship):		
With Dutch apple	1 oz.	31
With garden salad	1 oz.	30
With pineapple	1 oz.	35
Cream, plain, unwhipped:		
(Frigo)	1 oz.	100
Philadelphia (Kraft)	1 oz.	104
Edam:		
(House of Gold)	1 oz.	100
Laughing Cow	1 oz.	100
(Sargento)	1 oz.	101
Farmers:		
Dutch Garden Brand	1 oz.	100
(Friendship) regular or no salt added	1 oz.	40
(Sargento)	1 oz.	72
Wispride	1 oz.	100
Feta (Sargento) Danish, cups	1 oz.	76
Gjetost (Sargento) Norwegian	1 oz.	118
Gouda:		
(Frigo)	1 oz.	100
Laughing Cow, natural	1 oz.	110
(Sargento) baby, caraway or smoked	1 oz.	101
Wispride	1 oz.	100
Gruyere, *Swiss Knight*	1 oz.	100
Havarti (Sargento):		
Creamy	1 oz.	90
Creamy, 60% mild	1 oz.	117
Hot pepper (Sargento)	1 oz.	112
Jarlsberg (Sargento) Norwegian	1 oz.	100
Kettle Moraine (Sargento)	1 oz.	100
Limburger (Sargento) natural	1 oz.	93

Food and Description	Measure or Quantity	Calories
Monterey Jack:		
(Frigo)	1 oz.	100
(Sargento) Midget, Longhorn, shredded or sliced	1 oz.	106
Mozzarella:		
(Fisher) part skim milk	1 oz.	90
(Sargento):		
Bar, rounds, shredded, shredded with spices, sliced for pizza or square	1 oz.	79
Whole milk	1 oz.	100
Muenster:		
(Sargento) red rind	1 oz.	104
Wispride	1 oz.	100
Nibblin Curds (Sargento)	1 oz.	114
Parmesan:		
(Frigo):		
Grated	1 T.	23
Whole	1 oz.	110
(Sargento):		
Grated	1 T.	27
Wedge	1 oz.	110
Pizza (Sargento) shredded or sliced	1 oz.	90
Pot (Sargento) regular, French onion or garlic	1 oz.	30
Provolone:		
(Frigo)	1 oz.	90
Laughing Cow:		
Cube	⅙ oz.	12
Wedge	¾ oz.	55
(Sargento) sliced	1 oz.	100
Ricotta:		
(Frigo) part skim milk	1 oz.	43
(Sargento):		
Part skim milk	1 oz.	39
Whole milk	1 oz.	49
Romano (Sargento) wedge	1 oz.	110
Roquefort, natural	1 oz.	104
Samsoe (Sargento) Danish	1 oz.	101
Scamorze (Frigo)	1 oz.	79
Stirred Curd (Frigo)	1 oz.	110
String (Sargento)	1 oz.	90
Swiss:		
(Fisher) natural	1 oz.	100
(Frigo) domestic	1 oz.	100
(Sargento) domestic, or Finland, sliced	1 oz.	107
Taco (Sargento) shredded	1 oz.	105

Food and Description	Measure or Quantity	Calories
Washed curd (Frigo)	1 oz.	110
CHEESE FONDUE, *Swiss Knight*	1-oz. serving	60
CHEESE FOOD:		
American or cheddar:		
(Weight Watchers) colored or white	1-oz. slice	50
Wispride:		
Regular	1 oz.	90
& blue cheese	1 oz.	100
Hickory smoked	1 oz.	90
& port wine	1 oz.	100
Sharp	1 oz.	90
Cheez 'N Crackers (Kraft)	1 piece	127
Cheez-ola (Fisher)	1 oz.	90
Cracker Snack (Sargento)	1 oz.	90
Loaf, *Count Down* (Pauly)	1 oz.	40
Mun-chee (Pauly)	1 oz.	100
Pimiento (Pauly)	.8-oz. slice	73
Swiss (Pauly)	.8-oz. slice	74
CHEESE PUFFS, frozen (Durkee)	1 piece	59
CHEESE SPREAD:		
American or cheddar:		
(Fisher)	1 oz.	80
(Nabisco) *Snack Mate*	1 tsp.	16
Cheese 'n Bacon (Nabisco) *Snack Mate*	1 tsp.	16
Cheese Whiz (Kraft)	1 oz.	78
Count Down (Fisher)	1 oz.	30
Imitation (Fisher) *Chef's Delight*	1 oz.	40
Pimiento:		
(Nabisco) *Snack Mate*	1 tsp.	15
(Price's)	1 oz.	80
Sharp (Pauly)	.8 oz.	77
Swiss, process (Pauly)	.8 oz.	76
Velveeta (Kraft)	1 oz.	85
CHEESE STRAW, frozen (Durkee)	1 piece	29
CHENIN BLANC WINE (Inglenook)	3 fl. oz.	60
CHERRY, sweet:		
Fresh, with stems	½ cup	41
Canned, regular (Stokely-Van Camp) pitted, solids & liq.	½ cup	50
Canned, dietetic, solids & liq.:		
(Diet Delight) with pits, water pack	½ cup	70
(Featherweight) dark, water pack	½ cup	60
(Featherweight) light, water pack	½ cup	50
CHERRY, CANDIED	1 oz.	96

Food and Description	Measure or Quantity	Calories
CHERRY DRINK:		
Canned:		
(Hi-C)	6 fl. oz.	93
(Lincoln) cherry berry	6 fl. oz.	100
*Mix (Hi-C)	6 fl. oz.	72
***CHERRY HEERING** (Hiram Walker)	1 fl. oz.	80
CHERRY JELLY:		
Sweetened (Smucker's)	1 T.	53
Dietetic:		
(Featherweight)	1 T.	16
(Slenderella)	1 T.	24
CHERRY LIQUEUR (DeKuyper)	1 fl. oz.	75
Sweetened (Smucker's)	1 T.	53
Dietetic:		
(Dia-Mel)	1 tsp.	2
(Featherweight) imitation	1 T.	6
(S&W) *Nutradiet*, red, tart	1 T.	12
CHERRY SPREAD, low sugar		
(Smucker's)	1 T.	24
CHESTNUT, fresh, in shell	¼ lb.	220
CHEWING GUM:		
Sweetened:		
Bazooka, bubble	1¢ slice	18
Beechies, Chiclets, tiny dize	1 piece	6
Beech Nut; Beeman's; Big Red;		
Black Jack; Clove; Doublemint;		
Freedent; Fruit Punch; Juicy		
Fruit; Spearmint (Wrigley's);		
Teaberry	1 stick	10
Dentyne	1 piece	4
Dietetic:		
Bazooka, sugarless	1 piece	16
(Clark; *Care*Free*)	1 piece	7
(Estee) bubble or regular	1 piece	5
(Featherweight) bubble or regular	1 piece	4
CHEX, cereal (Ralston Purina):		
Rice	1 cup	110
Wheat	⅔ cup	110
Wheat & raisins	¾ cup	130
CHIANTI WINE:		
(Italian Swiss Colony)	3 fl. oz.	83
(Louis M. Martini)	3 fl. oz.	90
CHICKEN:		
Broiler, cooked, meat only	3 oz.	116
Fryer, fried, meat & skin	3 oz.	212
Fryer, fried, meat only	3 oz.	178

Food and Description	Measure or Quantity	Calories
Fryer, fried, a 2½ lb. chicken (weighed with bone before cooking) will give you:		
Back	1 back	139
Breast	½ breast	160
Leg or drumstick	1 leg	87
Neck	1 neck	127
Rib	1 rib	41
Thigh	1 thigh	122
Wing	1 wing	82
Fried skin	1 oz.	119
Hen & cock:		
Stewed, meat & skin	3 oz.	269
Stewed, dark meat only	3 oz.	176
Stewed, light meat only	3 oz.	153
Stewed, diced	½ cup	139
Roaster, roasted, dark or light meat without skin	3 oz.	156
CHICKEN À LA KING:		
Home recipe	1 cup	468
Canned (Swanson)	½ of 10½-oz. can	180
Frozen:		
(Banquet) *Cookin' Bag*	5-oz. pkg.	138
(Stouffer's) with rice	½ of 9½-oz. pkg.	165
(Weight Watcher's)	10-oz. bag	233
CHICKEN BOUILLON:		
(Herb-Ox):		
Cube	1 cube	6
Packet	1 packet	12
Low sodium (Featherweight)	1 tsp.	18
CHICKEN, BONED, CANNED:		
(Swanson) chunk:		
Mixin' chicken	2½ oz.	130
White	2½ oz.	110
Low sodium (Featherweight)	2½ oz.	154
CHICKEN, CREAMED, frozen (Stouffer's)	6½ oz.	300
CHICKEN DINNER OR ENTREE:		
Canned (Swanson) & dumplings	7½ oz.	220
Frozen:		
(Banquet):		
Regular:		
& dumplings	12-oz. dinner	282
Nuggets	12-oz. entree	932
Buffet Supper, & dumplings	2-lb. pkg.	1209
Man-Pleaser:		
& dressing	19-oz. dinner	713
Fried	17-oz. dinner	942

Food and Description	Measure or Quantity	Calories
(Green Giant):		
& broccoli with rice in cheese sauce	10-oz. entree	365
& pea pods in sauce with rice & vegetables	10-oz. entree	326
(Morton):		
Boneless	10-oz. dinner	222
Boneless, king size	17-oz. dinner	546
Country Table	15-oz. dinner	682
Country Table, fried	12-oz. entree	583
(Mrs. Paul's) pattie, breaded & fried with french fries	8½-oz. pkg.	389
(Stouffer's):		
Cacciatore, with spaghetti	11¼-oz. meal	313
Divan	8½-oz. serving	336
(Swanson):		
Regular, in white wine sauce	8¼-oz. entree	350
Hungry Man:		
Boneless	19-oz. dinner	680
Fried:		
White portion	15¼-oz. dinner	950
White portion with whipped potatoes	11¾-oz. entree	720
TV Brand, fried:		
Barbecue	11¼-oz. dinner	570
Nibbles, with french fries	6-oz. entree	380
3-course fried	15-oz. dinner	590
(Weight Watchers):		
New-Orleans style	11-oz. bag	229
Oriental style	12-oz. bag	251
Parmigiana, 2-compartment	7¾-oz. pkg.	220
Sliced, in celery sauce, 2-compartment	8½-oz. pkg.	207
Sliced, with gravy & stuffing, 3-compartment	14¾-oz. pkg.	380
Southern fried patty, 2-compartment	6¾-oz. serving	260
Sweet & sour	9½-oz. bag	220
CHICKEN, FRIED, frozen:		
(Banquet)	2-lb. pkg.	2591
(Morton)	2-lb. pkg.	1490
(Swanson):		
Assorted pieces	3¼-oz. serving	290
Breast	3¼-oz. serving	250
Nibbles (wing)	3¼-oz. serving	300
Take-out style	3¼-oz. serving	270
CHICKEN LIVER & ONION, frozen (Weight Watchers) 2-compartment	9¼-oz. meal	188

Food and Description	Measure or Quantity	Calories
CHICKEN LIVER PUFF, frozen		
(Durkee)	½-oz. piece	48
CHICKEN & NOODLES:		
Frozen:		
(Banquet) *Buffet Supper*	2-lb. pkg.	764
(Green Giant) with vegetables	9-oz. pkg.	365
(Stouffer's):		
Escalloped	5¾-oz. serving	252
Paprikash	10½-oz. serving	391
CHICKEN, PACKAGED (Louis Rich) breast, oven roasted	1-oz. slice	40
CHICKEN PIE, frozen:		
(Banquet) regular	8-oz. pie	427
(Morton)	8-oz. pie	345
(Stouffer's)	10-oz. pie	493
(Swanson):		
Regular	8-oz. pie	420
Hungry Man	1-lb. pie	730
(Van de Kamp's)	7½-oz. pie	520
CHICKEN PUFF (Durkee)	½-oz. piece	49
CHICKEN SALAD (Carnation)	1½-oz. serving	94
CHICKEN SOUP (See SOUP, Chicken)		
CHICKEN SPREAD:		
(Swanson)	1-oz. serving	60
(Underwood)	1-oz. serving	63
CHICKEN STEW, canned:		
Regular:		
(Libby's) with dumplings	8-oz. serving	194
(Swanson)	7⅝-oz. serving	170
Dietetic (Featherweight)	7¼-oz. can	170
CHICKEN STOCK BASE (French's)	1 tsp.	8
CHICK-FIL-A:		
Sandwich	5.4-oz. serving	404
Soup, hearty; breast of chicken:		
Small	8.5 oz.	131
Large	14.3 oz.	230
CHICK 'N QUICK, frozen (Tyson):		
Breast Fillet	3 oz.	210
Breast Pattie	3 oz.	240
Chick 'N Cheddar	3 oz.	250
Cordon bleu	5 oz.	300
Kiev	5 oz.	410
Swiss 'N Bacon	3 oz.	260
CHILI OR CHILI CON CARNE:		
Canned, regular pack:		
Beans only:		
(Blue Boy)	1 cup	290

Food and Description	Measure or Quantity	Calories
(Van Camp) Mexican style	1 cup	250
With beans:		
(Libby's)	½ of 15-oz. can	270
(Nalley's) mild or hot	8-oz. serving	314
(Swanson)	7¾-oz. serving	310
Without beans:		
(Libby's)	7½ oz.	390
(Nalley's) *Big Chunk*	7½-oz. can	383
Canned, dietetic pack		
(Featherweight) with beans	7½ oz.	270
Frozen, with beans (Weight Watchers) one-compartment	10-oz. pkg.	295
CHILI SAUCE:		
(Ortega) green	1 oz.	6
(Featherweight) dietetic	1 T.	8
CHILI SEASONING MIX:		
*(Durkee)	1 cup	465
(French's) *Chili-O*	2 pkg.	150
CHOCO-DILE (Hostess)	2-oz. piece	235
CHOCOLATE, BAKING:		
(Baker's):		
Bitter or unsweetened	1 oz.	180
Semi-sweet, chips	¼ cup	207
Sweetened, *German's*	1 oz.	158
(Hershey's):		
Bitter or unsweetened	1 oz.	188
Sweetened:		
Dark, chips, regular or mini	1 oz.	151
Milk, chips	1 oz.	148
Semi-sweet, chips	1 oz.	150
(Nestlé):		
Bitter or unsweetened, *Choco-Bake*	1-oz. packet	170
Sweet or semi-sweet, morsels	1 oz.	150
CHOCOLATE ICE CREAM (See ICE CREAM)		
CHOCOLATE SYRUP (See SYRUP, Chocolate)		
CHOP SUEY, frozen:		
(Banquet) beef:		
Buffet Supper	2-lb. pkg.	418
Cookin' Bag	7-oz. bag	73
Dinner	12-oz. dinner	282
(Stouffer's) beef, with rice	12-oz. pkg.	355
***CHOP SUEY SEASONING MIX**		
(Durkee)	1¾ cups	557
CHOWDER (See SOUP, Chowder)		

CHOW MEIN:
  Canned:
    (Chun King):

Food and Description	Measure or Quantity	Calories
Chicken	8-oz. serving	60
Pork, *Divider-Pak*	12-oz. serving	110
(Hormel) pork, *Short Orders*	7½-oz. can	140
(La Choy):		
Beef	1 cup	72
*Beef, bi-pack	1 cup	83
Chicken	½ of 1-lb. can	68
*Chicken, bi-pack	1 cup	101
Meatless	1 cup	47
*Mushroom, bi-pack	1 cup	85
Pepper Oriental	1 cup	89
*Pepper Oriental, bi-pack	1 cup	89
*Pork, bi-pack	1 cup	120
Shrimp	1 cup	61
*Shrimp, bi-pack	1 cup	110
Frozen:		
(Banquet)	12-oz. dinner	282
(Green Giant) chicken	9-oz. entree	215
(La Choy):		
Beef, 5-compartment	11-oz. dinner	337
Beef, entree	8-oz. serving	97
Chicken	11-oz. dinner	356
Pepper oriental	11-oz. dinner	332
Shrimp	11-oz. dinner	323
CHUTNEY (Major Grey's)	1 T.	53
CINNAMON, GROUND (French's)	1 tsp.	6
CITRUS COOLER DRINK, canned:		
(Hi-C)	6 fl. oz.	93
(Ann Page)	1 cup	
CLAM:		
Raw, all kinds, meat only	1 cup (8 oz.)	186
Raw, soft, meat & liq.	1 lb. (weighed in shell)	142
Canned (Doxsee):		
Chopped & minced, solids & liq.	4 oz.	59
Chopped, meat only	4 oz.	111
Frozen (Mrs. Paul's):		
Deviled	3-oz. piece	179
Fried	2½ oz.	264
CLAMATO COCKTAIL (Mott's)	6 fl. oz.	80
CLAM JUICE (Snow)	½ cup	15
CLAM SANDWICH, frozen (Mrs. Paul's) fried	4½-oz. sandwich	419
CLARET WINE:		
(Gold Seal)	3 fl. oz.	82

Food and Description	Measure or Quantity	Calories
(Inglenook) Navelle	3 fl. oz.	60
(Taylor) 12.5% alcohol	3 fl. oz.	72
CLORETS, gum or mint	1 piece	6
COCOA:		
Dry, unsweetened:		
(Hershey's)	1 T.	29
(Sultana)	1 T.	30
Mix, regular:		
(Alba '66) instant, all flavors	1 envelope	60
(Carnation) all flavors	1-oz. pkg.	112
(Hershey's):		
Hot	1 oz.	110
Instant	3 T.	76
(Nestlé):		
Hot	1 oz.	110
With mini marshmallows	1 oz.	110
(Ovaltine) hot 'n rich	1-oz. pkg.	120
Swiss Miss, regular or with mini marshmallows	6 fl. oz.	110
Mix, dietetic:		
(Carnation) *70 Calorie*	¾-oz. packet	70
*(Featherweight)	6 fl. oz.	50
(Ovaltine) hot, reduced calorie	.45-oz. pkg.	50
Swiss Miss, instant, lite	3 T.	70
COCOA KRISPIES, cereal (Kellogg's)	¾ cup	110
COCOA PUFFS, cereal (General Mills)	1 oz.	110
COCONUT:		
Fresh, meat only	2″ × 2″ × ½″ piece	156
Grated or shredded, loosely packed	½ cup	225
Dried:		
(Baker's):		
Angel Flake	⅓ cup	118
Cookie	⅓ cup	186
Premium shred	⅓ cup	138
(Durkee) shredded	¼ cup	69
COCO WHEATS, cereal	1 T.	44
COD, broiled	3 oz.	145
COFFEE:		
Regular:		
*Max-Pax; Maxwell House Electra Perk; Yuban; Yuban Electra Matic	6 fl. oz.	2
*Mellow Roast	6 fl. oz.	8
Decaffeinated:		
*Brim, regular or electric perk	6 fl. oz.	2
*Brim, freeze-dried; Decafé; Nescafé	6 fl. oz.	4

Food and Description	Measure or Quantity	Calories
*Sanka, regular or electric perk	6 fl. oz.	2
*Freeze-dried, Maxim, Sanka, Taster's Choice	6 fl. oz.	4
Instant:		
*(Chase & Sanborn)	5 fl. oz.	1
*Decaf (Nestlé); Nescafé	6 fl. oz.	4
*Mellow Roast	6 fl. oz.	8
*Sunrise	6 fl. oz.	6
*Mix (General Foods) International Coffee:		
Cafe Amaretto, Cafe Francais	6 fl. oz.	59
Cafe Vienna, Orange Capuccino	6 fl. oz.	65
Irish Mocha Mint	6 fl. oz.	55
Suisse Mocha	6 fl. oz.	58
COFFEE CAKE (See CAKE, Coffee)		
COFFEE LIQUEUR (DeKuyper)	1½ fl. oz.	140
COFFEE SOUTHERN	1 fl. oz.	79
COLA SOFT DRINK (See SOFT DRINK, Cola)		
COLD DUCK WINE (Great Western) pink	3 fl. oz.	92
COLESLAW, solids & liq., made with mayonnaise-type salad dressing	1 cup	119
***COLESLAW MIX** (Libby's) Super Slaw	½ cup	240
COLLARDS:		
Leaves, cooked	½ cup	31
Canned (Sunshine) chopped, solids & liq.	½ cup	25
Frozen:		
(Birds Eye) chopped	⅓ pkg.	31
(McKenzie) chopped	⅓ pkg.	25
(Southland) chopped	⅕ of 16-oz. pkg.	30
COMPLETE CEREAL (Elam's)	1 oz.	109
CONCORD WINE:		
(Gold Seal)	3 fl. oz.	125
(Mogen David)	3 fl. oz.	120
(Pleasant Valley) red	3 fl. oz.	90
COOKIE, REGULAR:		
Almond Windmill (Nabisco)	1 piece	47
Animal:		
(Dixie Belle)	1 piece	8
(Keebler):		
Regular	1 piece	12
Iced	1 piece	24
(Nabisco) Barnum's Animals	1 piece	12
(Ralston)		
Apple (Pepperidge Farm)	1 piece	50

Food and Description	Measure or Quantity	Calories
Apple Crisp (Nabisco)	1 piece	50
Apple Spice (Pepperidge Farm)	1 piece	53
Apricot Raspberry (Pepperidge Farm)	1 piece	50
Assortment:		
(Nabisco) *Mayfair*:		
Crown creme sandwich	1 piece	53
Fancy shortbread biscuit	1 piece	22
Filigree creme sandwich	1 piece	60
Mayfair creme sandwich	1 piece	65
Tea rose creme	1 piece	53
(Pepperidge Farm):		
Butter	1 piece	55
Champagne	1 piece	32
Chocolate lace & Pirouette	1 piece	37
Marseilles	1 piece	45
Seville	1 piece	55
Southport	1 piece	75
Bordeaux (Pepperidge Farm)	1 piece	33
Brown edge wafers (Nabisco)	1 piece	28
Brownie:		
(Hostess)	1¼-oz. piece	157
(Pepperidge Farm) chocolate nut	.4-oz. cookie	57
(Sara Lee) frozen	⅛ of 13-oz. pkg.	199
Brussels (Pepperidge Farm)	1 piece	53
Brussels Mint (Pepperidge Farm)	1 piece	67
Butter (Nabisco)	1 piece	23
Cappucino (Pepperidge Farm)	1 piece	53
Caramel peanut log (Nabisco) *Heyday*	1 piece	120
Chessman (Pepperidge Farm)	1 piece	43
Chocolate & chocolate-covered:		
(Nabisco):		
Famous wafer	1 piece	28
Pinwheel, cake	1 piece	140
Snap	1 piece	16
Chocolate chip:		
(Keebler) *Rich 'N Chips*	1 piece	81
(Nabisco):		
Chips Ahoy!	1 piece	53
Chocolate	1 piece	53
Cookie Little	1 piece	7
(Pepperidge Farm):		
Regular size	1 piece	50
Large	1 piece	130
Coconut:		
(Keebler) chocolate drop	1 piece	83
(Nabisco) bar, *Bakers Bonus*	1 piece	43

44

Food and Description	Measure or Quantity	Calories
Coconut Granola (Pepperidge Farm)	1 piece	57
Creme Stick (Dutch Twin) chocolate coated	1 piece	39
Date Nut Granola (Pepperidge Farm)	1 piece	53
Fig bar:		
(Keebler)	1 piece	74
(Nabisco):		
Fig Newtons	1 piece	60
Fig Wheats	1 piece	60
Gingerman (Pepperidge Farm)	1 piece	57
Gingersnaps (Nabisco) old fashioned	1 piece	30
Granola (Pepperidge Farm) large	1 piece	120
Hazelnut (Pepperidge Farm)	1 piece	57
Ladyfinger	3¼″ × 1 ⅜″ × 1 ⅛″	40
Lemon Nut (Pepperidge Farm) large	1 piece	140
Lido (Pepperidge Farm)	1 piece	95
Macaroon, coconut (Nabisco)	1 piece	95
Marshmallow:		
(Nabisco):		
Mallomars	1 piece	60
Puffs, cocoa covered	1 piece	85
Sandwich	1 piece	30
Twirls cakes	1 piece	130
(Planters) banana pie	1 oz.	127
Milano (Pepperidge Farm)	1 piece	60
Mint Milano (Pepperidge Farm)	1 piece	76
Molasses (Nabisco) *Pantry*	1 piece	60
Molasses Crisp (Pepperidge Farm)	1 piece	33
Nilla wafer (Nabisco)	1 piece	19
Oatmeal:		
(Keebler) old fashion	1 piece	83
(Nabisco):		
Bakers Bonus	1 piece	80
Cookie Little	1 piece	6
(Pepperidge Farm):		
Irish	1 piece	47
Large	1 piece	120
Orange Milano (Pepperidge Farm)	1 piece	76
Peanut & peanut butter (Nabisco):		
Biscos	1 piece	47
Creme pattie	1 piece	35
Fudge	1 piece	50
Nutter Butter	1 piece	70
Peanut brittle (Nabisco)	1 piece	50
Pecan Sandies (Keebler)	1 piece	86
Raisin	1 oz.	107

45

Food and Description	Measure or Quantity	Calories
Raisin (Nabisco) fruit biscuit	1 piece	60
Raisin bar (Keebler) iced	1 piece	80
Raisin Bran (Pepperidge Farm)	1 piece	53
Sandwich:		
(Keebler):		
Chocolate fudge	1 piece	83
Elfwich	1 piece	55
Pitter Patter	1 piece	83
(Nabisco):		
Cameo creme	1 piece	70
Mystic mint	1 piece	90
OREO	1 piece	50
Oreo, double stuff	1 piece	70
Vanilla, *Cookie Break*	1 piece	50
Shortbread or shortcake:		
(Nabisco):		
Cookie Little	1 piece	6
Lorna Doone	1 piece	40
Melt-A-Way	1 piece	70
Pecan	1 piece	80
(Pepperidge Farm)	1 piece	75
Social Tea, biscuit (Nabisco)	1 piece	22
Spiced wafers (Nabisco)	1 piece	33
Spiced Windmill (Keebler)	1 piece	60
Sugar cookie (Nabisco) rings, *Bakers Bonus*	1 piece	70
Sugar wafer:		
(Dutch Twin) any flavor	1 piece	36
(Keebler) *Krisp Kreem*	1 piece	29
(Nabisco) *Biscos*	1 piece	19
Sunflower Raisin (Pepperidge Farm)	1 piece	53
Tahiti (Pepperidge Farm)	1 piece	85
Vanilla creme (Planters)	1 oz.	116
Vanilla wafer (Keebler)	1 piece	19
Waffle creme (Dutch Twin)	1 piece	45
Zanzibar (Pepperidge Farm)	1 piece	40
COOKIE, DIETETIC (Estee):		
Chocolate chip	1 piece	28
Coconut	1 piece	25
Fudge	1 piece	27
Oatmeal Raisin	1 piece	23
Sandwich duplex	1 piece	47
Wafer, chocolate covered	1 piece	128
COOKIE CRISP, cereal, any flavor	1 cup	110
***COOKIE DOUGH:**		
Refrigerated (Pillsbury):		
Chocolate chip	1 cookie	53
Oatmeal or peanut butter	1 cookie	57

Food and Description	Measure or Quantity	Calories
Sugar	1 cookie	60
Frozen (Rich's):		
Chocolate chip	1 cookie	138
Oatmeal	1 cookie	125
Sugar	1 cookie	118
*COOKIE MIX:		
Regular:		
Brownie:		
(Betty Crocker):		
Fudge, regular style	1/16 of pan	150
Walnut, family size	1/24 of pan	130
(Nestlé)	1/23 of pkg.	150
(Pillsbury) fudge, regular size	1½" square (1/36 pkg.)	65
Chocolate chip:		
(Betty Crocker) *Big Batch*	1 cookie	60
(Duncan Hines)	1/36 of pkg.	72
(Nestlé)	1 cookie	60
(Quaker)	1 cookie	75
Fudge chip (Quaker)	1 cookie	75
Macaroon, coconut		
(Betty Crocker)	1/24 of pkg.	80
Oatmeal:		
(Betty Crocker) *Big Batch*	1 cookie	65
(Duncan Hines) raisin	1/36 of pkg.	68
(Nestlé) raisin	1 cookie	60
(Quaker)	1 cookie	66
Peanut butter (Duncan Hines)	1/36 pkg.	68
Sugar:		
(Betty Crocker) *Big Batch*	1 cookie	60
(Duncan Hines) golden	1/36 of pkg.	59
Dietetic (Dia-Mel)	2" cookie	50
COOKING SPRAY, *Mazola No Stick*	2-second spray	8
CORN:		
Fresh, on the cob, boiled	5" × 1¾" ear	70
Canned, regular pack:		
(Del Monte):		
Cream style, golden, wet pack	4¼ oz.	95
Whole kernel, drained	4 oz.	100
Whole kernel, vacuum pack	4 oz.	101
(Festal):		
Cream style, golden, wet pack	½ cup	89
Golden, whole kernel, drained	½ pan	100
(Green Giant):		
Cream style	4¼ oz.	96
Whole kernel, solids & liq.	4¼ oz.	79
Whole kernel, *Mexicorn,* solids & liq.	3½ oz.	90

Food and Description	Measure or Quantity	Calories
(Libby's):		
Cream style	½ cup	100
Whole kernel, solids & liq.	½ cup	92
(Stokely-Van Camp):		
Cream style	½ cup	105
Whole kernel, solids & liq.	½ cup	74
Canned, dietetic pack:		
(Diet Delight) solids & liq.	½ cup	60
(Featherweight) whole kernel, solids & liq.	½ cup	80
(S&W) *Nutradiet*, solids & liq.	½ cup	80
Frozen:		
(Birds Eye):		
On the cob:		
Farmside	4.4-oz. ear	140
Little Ears	2.3-oz. ear	73
Jubilee	⅓ of pkg.	118
Whole kernel	⅓ of pkg.	96
(Green Giant):		
On the cob	5½" ear	133
On the cob, *Nibbler*	3" ear	73
Whole kernel, *Harvest Fresh*	4 oz.	101
Whole kernel, *Niblets*, golden, in butter sauce	⅓ of pkg.	85
Whole kernel, white, in butter sauce	⅓ of pkg.	87
(McKenzie) on the cob	5" ear	120
(Seabrook Farms):		
On the cob	5" ear	140
Whole kernel	⅓ of pkg.	97
CORNBREAD:		
Home recipe:		
Corn pone	4 oz.	231
Spoon bread	4 oz.	221
*Mix:		
(Aunt Jemima)	⅙ of pkg.	220
(Dromedary)	2" × 2" piece	130
(Pillsbury) *Ballard*	⅛ of recipe	140
*CORN DOGS, frozen, (Oscar Mayer)	4-oz. piece	328
CORNED BEEF:		
Cooked, boneless, medium fat	4 oz.	422
Canned:		
Dinty Moore	3-oz. serving	196
(Libby's)	⅓ of 7-oz. can	160
Dietetic (Featherweight) loaf	2½ oz.	90
Packaged:		
(Eckrich) sliced	1-oz. slice	41

Food and Description	Measure or Quantity	Calories
(Oscar Mayer) jellied loaf (Vienna):	1-oz. slice	44
Brisket	1-oz. serving	88
Flats	1-oz. serving	49
(Libby's)	⅓ of 24-oz. can	420
Mary Kitchen	7½-oz. serving	399
CORNED BEEF HASH DINNER, frozen (Banquet)	10-oz. dinner	372
CORNED BEEF SPREAD (Underwood)	1 oz.	53
CORN FLAKE CRUMBS (Kellogg's)	¼ cup	110
CORN FLAKES, cereal:		
(Featherweight) low sodium	1¼ cups	110
(General Mills) *Country*	1 cup	110
(Kellogg's)	1 cup	110
(Kellogg's) honey & nut	¾ cup	120
(Post) *Post Toasties*	1¼ cups	107
(Ralston Purina) regular or sugar frosted	1 cup	110
(Van Brode) regular	1 oz.	107
CORN MEAL:		
Bolted (Aunt Jemima/Quaker)	3 T.	102
Degermed	¼ cup	125
Mix:		
Bolted (Aunt Jemima)	1 cup	392
Degermed (Aunt Jemima)	1 cup	392
CORNNUTS	1-oz. serving	120
CORNSTARCH (Argo: Kingsford's; Duryea)	1 tsp.	11
CORN SYRUP (See SYRUP)		
COUGH DROP:		
(Beech-Nut)	1 drop	10
(Pine Bros.)	1 drop	8
(Smith Brothers)	1 drop	7
COUNT CHOCULA, cereal (General Mills)	1 oz. (1 cup)	110
CRAB:		
Fresh, steamed:		
Whole	½ lb.	101
Meat only	4 oz.	105
Canned, king crab (Icy Point; Pillar Rock)	3¾ oz.	108
Frozen (Wakefield's Alaska King)	4 oz.	96
CRAB APPLE	¼ lb.	71
CRAB APPLE JELLY (Smucker's)	1 T.	53
CRAB, DEVILED, breaded & fried (Mrs. Paul's) regular	½ of 6-oz. pkg.	154
CRAB IMPERIAL, home recipe	1 cup	323

Food and Description	Measure or Quantity	Calories
CRACKED WHEAT CEREAL		
(Elam's)	1 oz.	100
CRACKER PUFFS & CHIPS:		
Arrowroot biscuit (Nabisco)	1 piece	20
Bacon 'n Dip (Nabisco)	1 piece	21
Bacon-flavored thins (Nabisco)	1 piece	11
Bacon Nips	1 oz.	147
Bacon Toast (Keebler)	1 piece	16
Biscos (Nabisco)	1 piece	19
Bran Wafer (Featherweight)	1 piece	13
Bugles (General Mills)	1 oz.	150
Cheese Flavored:		
Bops (Nalley's)	1 oz.	147
Cheddar Bitz (Frito-Lay)	1 oz.	129
Cheddar triangles (Nabisco)	1 piece	9
Cheese 'n Crunch (Nabisco)	1 oz.	160
Cheese Pixies (Wise) baked	1 oz.	155
Chee.Tos, crunchy	1 oz.	160
Chee.Tos, puffed	1 oz.	160
Cheez Balls (Planters)	1 oz.	160
Cheez Curls (Planters)	1 oz.	160
Country cheddar'n sesame (Nabisco)	1 piece	9
Nacho cheese cracker (Keebler)	1 piece	11
(Ralston)	1 piece	6
Swiss cheese (Nabisco)	1 piece	10
Tid-Bit (Nabisco)	1 oz.	150
Twists (Bachman) baked	1 oz.	150
Chicken in a Biskit (Nabisco)	1 piece	11
Chip O'Cheddar, Flavor Kist, (Schulze and Burch)	1 oz.	130
Chippers (Nabisco)	1 piece	15
Chipsters (Nabisco)	1 piece	2
Club cracker (Keebler)	1 piece	15
Corn chips:		
(Bachman) regular or BBQ	1 oz.	150
(Featherweight) low sodium	1 oz.	170
Fritos	1 oz.	160
Fritos, barbecue flavor	1 oz.	150
Korkers (Nabisco)	1 piece	8
Corn Nuts (Nalley's)	1 oz.	120
Corn & Sesame Chips (Nabisco)	1 piece	10
Creme Wafer Stock (Nabisco)	1 piece	47
Crown Pilot (Nabisco)	1 piece	75
Diggers (Nabisco)	1 piece	4
Dixies (Nabisco)	1 piece	8
English Water Biscuit (Pepperidge Farm)	1 piece	17

Food and Description	Measure or Quantity	Calories
Escort (Nabisco)	1 piece	21
French onion cracker (Nabisco)	1 piece	12
Goldfish (Pepperidge Farm):		
Thins	1 piece	10
Tiny	1 piece	3
Graham:		
Cinnamon Treat (Nabisco)	1 piece	28
(Dixie Belle) sugar-honey coated	1 piece	15
Flavor Kist (Schulze and Burch)		
sugar-honey coated	1 piece	57
Honey Maid (Nabisco)	1 piece	30
Graham, chocolate or		
cocoa-covered:		
Fancy Dip (Nabisco)	1 piece	65
(Keebler)	1 piece	43
(Nabisco)	1 piece	57
Lil' Loaf (Nabisco)	1 piece	14
Melba Toast (See MELBA TOAST)		
Milk Lunch Biscuit (Keebler)	1 piece	27
Mucho Macho Nacho, Flavor Kist,		
(Schulze and Burch)	1 oz.	121
Oyster:		
(Keebler) *Zesta*	1 piece	2
(Nabisco) *Dandy* or *Oysterettes*	1 piece	3
Pumpernickel Toast (Keebler)	1 piece	15
Ritz (Nabisco)	1 piece	17
Roman Meal Wafer, boxed	1 piece	11
Royal Lunch (Nabisco)	1 piece	55
Rusk, *Holland* (Nabisco)	1 piece	40
Rye Toast (Keebler)	1 piece	16
Ry-Krisp, natural	1 triple cracker	25
Ry-Krisp, seasoned or sesame	1 triple cracker	30
Rye wafers (Nabisco)	1 piece	23
Saltine:		
(Dixie Belle) regular or unsalted	1 piece	12
Flavor Kist (Schulze and Burch)	1 piece	12
Premium (Nabisco)	1 piece	12
Zesta (Keebler)	1 piece	13
Sea Toast (Keebler)	1 piece	60
Sesame:		
Butter flavored (Nabisco)	1 piece	17
Sesame Wheats! (Nabisco)	1 piece	17
Sesame wheat snack, *Flavor Kist*		
(Schulze and Burch)	1 oz.	134
Teeko (Nabisco)	1 piece	22
Toast (Keebler)	1 piece	15
Shindigs (Keebler)	1 piece	6
Skittle Chips (Nabisco)	1 piece	14

Food and Description	Measure or Quantity	Calories
Snackers (Ralston)	1 piece	17
Snackin' Crisp (Durkee) *O & C*	1 oz.	155
Snacks Sticks (Pepperidge Farm):		
Cheese	1 piece	17
Lightly salted, pumpernickel, rye & sesame	1 piece	16
Table Water Cracker (Carr's) small	1 piece	15
Tater Puffs (Nabisco)	1 piece	7
Tortillo chips:		
(Bachman) nacho, taco flavor or toasted	1 oz.	140
Buenos (Nabisco) nacho flavor	1 piece	10
Doritos, nacho or taco flavor	1 oz.	140
(Nabisco) regular and nacho flavor	1 piece	11
(Nalley's)	1 oz.	147
(Planters) nacho or taco flavor	1 oz.	130
Tostitos	1 oz.	140
Town House Cracker (Keebler)	1 piece	16
Triscuit (Nabisco)	1 piece	20
Twigs (Nabisco)	1 piece	14
Uneeda Biscuit (Nabisco) unsalted	1 piece	22
Unsalted (Featherweight)	2 sections (½ cracker)	30
Waldorf (Keebler) low sodium	1 piece	14
Waverly Wafer (Nabisco)	1 piece	18
Wheat (Pepperidge Farm) cracked or hearty	1 piece	28
Wheat Chips (Nabisco)	1 piece	4
Wheat Crisps (Keebler)	1 piece	13
Wheatmeal Biscuit (Carr's) small	1 piece	42
Wheat Snack (Dixie Belle)	1 piece	9
Wheat snack, *Flavor Kist* (Schulze and Burch):		
Regular	1 oz.	138
Rye	1 oz.	130
Wild onion	1 oz.	125
Wheatsworth (Nabisco)	1 piece	14
Wheat Thins (Nabisco)	1 piece	9
Wheat Toast (Keebler)	1 piece	15
Wheat wafer (Featherweight) unsalted	1 piece	13
CRACKER CRUMBS, graham (Nabisco)	⅛ of 9″ pie shell	70
CRACKER MEAL (Nabisco)	½ cup	220
CRANAPPLE JUICE (Ocean Spray) canned:		
Regular	6 fl. oz.	129
Dietetic	6 fl. oz.	32

Food and Description	Measure or Quantity	Calories
CRANBERRY, fresh (Ocean Spray)	½ cup	26
*CRANBERRY-APPLE JUICE, frozen (Welch's)	6 fl. oz.	120
*CRANBERRY-GRAPE JUICE, frozen (Welch's)	6 fl. oz.	110
*CRANBERRY JUICE COCKTAIL:		
Canned (Ocean Spray):		
Regular	6 fl. oz.	106
Dietetic	6 fl. oz.	36
*Frozen (Welch's)	6 fl. oz.	100
CRANBERRY-ORANGE JUICE DRINK (Ocean Spray)	6 fl. oz.	101
CRANBERRY-ORANGE RELISH (Ocean Spray)	1 T.	33
CRANBERRY-RASPBERRY SAUCE (Ocean Spray) jellied	2-oz. serving	85
CRANBERRY SAUCE:		
Home recipe	4 oz.	202
Canned (Ocean Spray):		
Jellied	2-oz. serving	88
Whole berry	2-oz. serving	89
CRANGRAPE (Ocean Spray)	6 fl. oz.	108
*CRANORANGE JUICE DRINK, frozen (Ocean Spray)	6 fl. oz.	107
CRAN-RASPBERRY SAUCE (Ocean Spray) jellied	2-oz. serving	89
CRAZY COW, cereal (General Mills)	1 cup	110
CREAM:		
Half & Half (Dairylea)	1 fl. oz.	40
Light, table or coffee (Sealtest) 16% fat	1 T.	26
Light, whipping, 30% fat (Sealtest)	1 T.	45
Heavy whipping (Dairylea)	1 fl. oz.	60
Sour (Dairylea)	1 fl. oz.	60
Sour, imitation (Pet)	1 T.	25
Substitute (See CREAM SUBSTITUTE)		
CREAM PUFFS:		
Home recipe, custard filling	3½″ × 2″ piece	303
Frozen (Rich's) chocolate	1⅓-oz. piece	146
CREAMSICLE (Popsicle Industries)	2½-fl. oz. piece	80
CREAM SUBSTITUTE:		
Coffee Mate (Carnation)	1 tsp.	11
Coffee Rich	½ oz.	22
Coffee Twin	½ fl. oz.	18
Dairy Light (Alba)	2.8-oz. envelope	10
N-Rich	1½ tsp.	15
Perx	1 tsp.	8

Food and Description	Measure or Quantity	Calories
(Pet)	1 tsp.	10
CREAM OF WHEAT, cereal:		
*Instant	¾ cup	100
Mix'n Eat, dry:		
Regular	1 packet	100
Baked apple & cinnamon	1 packet	130
Banana & spice	1 packet	130
Maple & brown sugar	3¾ T.	130
Quick	2½ T.	100
Regular	2½ T.	100
CREME DE BANANA LIQUEUR		
(Mr. Boston)	1 fl. oz.	93
CREME DE CACAO:		
(Garnier)	1 fl. oz.	97
(Hiram Walker)	1 fl. oz.	104
(Mr. Boston):		
Brown	1 fl. oz.	103
White	1 fl. oz.	93
CREME DE CASSIS:		
(Garnier)	1 fl. oz.	83
(Mr. Boston)	1 fl. oz.	85
CREME DE MENTHE:		
(Bols)	1 fl. oz.	122
(Hiram Walker)	1 fl. oz.	94
(Mr. Boston):		
Green	1 fl. oz.	109
White	1 fl. oz.	97
CREME DE NOYAUX (Mr. Boston)	1 fl. oz.	99
CREPE, frozen:		
(Mrs. Paul's):		
Crab	5½-oz. pkg.	248
Shrimp	5½-oz. pkg.	252
(Stouffer's):		
Beef burgundy	6¼-oz. pkg.	335
Chicken with mushroom sauce	8¼-oz. pkg.	390
Mushroom	6¼-oz. pkg.	255
CRISP RICE, cereal:		
(Featherweight) low sodium	1 cup	110
(Ralston Purina)	1 cup	110
(Van Brode)	1 cup	107
CRISPY WHEATS 'N RAISINS, cereal (General Mills)	¾ cup	110
CROQUETTES, frozen, seafood (Mrs. Paul's)	3-oz. serving	181
CROUTON:		
(Arnold):		
Bavarian or English style	½ oz.	65
French, Italian or Mexican style	½ oz.	66

Food and Description	Measure or Quantity	Calories
(Kellogg's) *Croutettes*	⅔ cup	70
(Pepperidge Farm):		
Cheddar & romano	.5 oz.	60
Cheese & garlic or seasoned	.5 oz.	70
CUCUMBER:		
Eaten with skin	½-lb. cucumber	32
Pared, 10-oz. cucumber	7½″ × 2″ pared	29
Pared	3 slices	4
CUMIN SEED (French's)	1 tsp.	7
CUPCAKE:		
Regular (Hostess):		
Chocolate	1 cupcake	166
Orange	1 cupcake	151
Frozen (Sara Lee) yellow	1 cupcake	190
*****CUPCAKE MIX** (Flako)	1 cupcake	150
CUP O'NOODLES (Nissin Foods):		
Beef	2½-oz. serving	343
Beef, twin pack	1.2-oz. serving	151
Beef onion	2½-oz. serving	323
Beef onion, twin pack	1.2-oz. serving	158
Chicken	2½-oz. serving	343
Chicken, twin pack	1.2-oz. serving	155
Pork	2½-oz. serving	331
Shrimp	2½-oz. serving	336
CURAÇAO:		
(Bols)	1 fl. oz.	105
(Hiram Walker)	1 fl. oz.	96
CURRANT, dried, Zante (Del Monte)	½ cup	204
CURRANT JELLY (Smucker's)	1 T.	53
CUSTARD:		
Chilled, *Swiss Miss*, chocolate or egg flavor	4-oz. container	150
*****Mix, dietetic (Featherweight)	½ cup	80
C.W. POST, cereal:		
Plain	¼ cup	131
With raisins	¼ cup	128

D

DAIRY QUEEN/BRAZIER:		
Banana split	13.5-oz. serving	540
Brownie Delight, hot fudge	9.4-oz. serving	600
Buster Bar	5¼-oz. piece	460
Chicken sandwich	7.76-oz. sandwich	670

Food and Description	Measure or Quantity	Calories
Cone:		
Plain, any flavor:		
Small	3-oz. cone	140
Regular	5-oz. cone	240
Large	7½-oz. cone	340
Dipped, chocolate:		
Small	3¼-oz. cone	190
Regular	5½-oz. cone	340
Large	8¼-oz. cone	510
Dilly Bar	3-oz. piece	210
Double Delight	9-oz. service†	490
DQ sandwich	2.1-oz. serving	140
Fish sandwich:		
Plain	6-oz. sandwich	400
With cheese	6.24-oz. sandwich	440
Float	14-oz. serving	410
Freeze, vanilla	14-oz. serving	500
French fries:		
Regular	2½-oz. serving	200
Large	4-oz. serving	320
Frozen dessert	4-oz. serving	180
Hamburger:		
Plain:		
Single	5.2-oz. sandwich	360
Double	7.4-oz. sandwich	530
Triple	9.6-oz. sandwich	710
With cheese:		
Single	5.7-oz. sandwich	410
Double	8.43-oz. sandwich	650
Triple	10.62-oz. sandwich	820
Hot dog:		
Regular:		
Plain	3.53-oz. serving	280
With cheese	4-oz. serving	330
With chili	4½-oz. serving	320
Super:		
Plain	6.2-oz. serving	520
With cheese	6.9-oz. serving	580
With chili	7.7-oz. serving	570
Lettuce	½ oz.	2
Malt, chocolate:		
Small	10.26-oz. serving	520
Regular	14.74-oz. serving	760
Large	20.74-oz. serving	1060
Mr. Misty:		
Plain:		
Small	8¾-oz. serving	190
Regular	11.64-oz. serving	250

Food and Description	Measure or Quantity	Calories
Large	15.5-oz. serving	340
Kiss	3.14-oz. serving	70
Float	14½-oz. serving	390
Freeze	14½-oz. serving	500
Onion rings	3-oz.	280
Parfait	10 oz.	430
Peanut Butter Parfait	10¾-oz. serving	740
Shake, chocolate:		
Small	10¼-oz. serving	490
Regular	14¾-oz. serving	710
Large	20¾-oz. serving	990
Strawberry shortcake	11 oz.	540
Sundae, chocolate:		
Small	3¾-oz. serving	190
Regular	6¼-oz. serving	310
Large	8¾-oz. serving	440
Tomato	½ oz.	4
DAIQUIRI COCKTAIL, canned (Mr. Boston):		
Regular	3 fl. oz.	99
Strawberry	3 fl. oz.	111
DATE (Dromedary):		
Chopped	¼ cup	130
Pitted	5 dates	100
DE CHAUNAC WINE (Great Western) 12% alcohol	3 fl. oz.	71
DELAWARE WINE (Gold Seal) 12% alcohol	3 fl. oz.	87
DELI's frozen (Pepperidge Farm):		
Beef with barbecue sauce	4-oz. piece	270
Mexican style	4-oz. piece	280
Reuben in rye pastry	4-oz. piece	360
Savory chicken salad	4-oz. piece	340
Turkey, ham & cheese	4-oz. piece	270
DESSERT CUPS (Hostess)	¾-oz. piece	62
DILL SEED (French's)	1 tsp.	9
DING DONG (Hostess)	1 cake	172
DINNER, frozen (See individual listings such as BEEF, CHICKEN, TURKEY, etc.)		
DIP:		
Avocado (Nalley's)	1 oz.	114
Barbecue (Nalley's)	1 oz.	114
Blue cheese:		
(Dean) tang	1 oz.	61
(Nalley's)	1 oz.	110
Clam (Nalley's)	1 oz.	101
Cucumber & onion (Breakstone)	1 oz.	50

Food and Description	Measure or Quantity	Calories
Enchilada, *Fritos*	1 oz.	37
Garlic (Nalley's)	1 oz.	120
Guacamole (Nalley's)	1 oz.	114
Jalapeno:		
Fritos	1 oz.	34
(Hain) natural	1 oz.	40
Onion (Dean) French	1 oz.	58
Onion bean (Hain) natural	1 oz.	41
DISTILLED LIQUOR, any brand:		
80 proof	1 fl. oz.	65
86 proof	1 fl. oz.	70
90 proof	1 fl. oz.	74
94 proof	1 fl. oz.	77
100 proof	1 fl. oz.	83
DONUTZ, cereal (General Mills)	1 cup	120
DOUGHNUT (See also *WINCHELL'S*):		
Regular (Hostess):		
Chocolate coated	1-oz. piece	137
Cinnamon	1-oz. piece	114
Donettes, frosted	1 piece	58
Old fashioned, plain	1½-oz. piece	179
Powdered	1-oz. piece	120
Frozen (Morton):		
Boston creme	2.3-oz. piece	208
Chocolate iced	1½-oz. piece	148
Jelly	1.8-oz. piece	175
DRAMBUIE (Hiram Walker)	1 fl. oz.	110
DRUMSTICK, frozen:		
Ice Cream, in a cone:		
Topped with peanuts	1 piece	181
Topped with peanuts & cone bisque	1 piece	168
Ice Milk, in a cone:		
Topped with peanuts	1 piece	163
Topped with peanuts & cone bisque	1 piece	150
DUMPLINGS, canned, dietetic (Featherweight)	7½ oz.	160

E

ECLAIR:		
Home recipe, with custard filling and chocolate icing	4-oz. piece	271

Frozen (Rich's) chocolate	1 piece	234
EEL, smoked, meat only	4 oz.	374
EGG, CHICKEN:		
Raw, white only	1 large egg	17
Raw, yolk only	1 large egg	59
Boiled	1 large egg	81
Fried in butter	1 large egg	99
Omelet, mixed with milk & cooked in fat	1 large egg	107
Poached	1 large egg	78
Scrambled, mixed with milk & cooked in fat	1 large egg	111
*EGG FOO YOUNG (Chun King) stir fry	⅙ of pkg.	45
EGG MIX (Durkee):		
Omelet:		
*With bacon	½ of pkg.	310
*Puffy	½ of pkg.	302
Scrambled:		
Plain	.8-oz. pkg.	124
With bacon	1.3-oz. pkg.	181
EGG NOG, dairy (Meadow Gold) 6% fat	½ cup	164
EGG NOG COCKTAIL (Mr. Boston) 15% alcohol	3 fl. oz.	180
EGGPLANT:		
Boiled	4 oz.	22
Frozen:		
(Mrs. Paul's):		
Parmesan	5½-oz. serving	259
Slices, breaded & fried	3-oz. serving	235
Sticks, breaded & fried	3½-oz. serving	262
(Weight Watchers) parmigiana	13-oz. pkg.	285
EGG ROLL, frozen:		
(Chun King):		
Chicken	½-oz. roll	23
Shrimp	½-oz. roll	23
(La Choy):		
Chicken	.4-oz. roll	30
Lobster	.4-oz. roll	27
Meat & shrimp	.2-oz. roll	17
Shrimp	2½-oz. roll	108
EGG, SCRAMBLED, frozen (Swanson) and sausage with hashed brown potatoes, *TV Brand*	6½-oz. entree	430
EGG SUBSTITUTE:		
Egg Magic (Featherweight)	½ envelope	60
*Eggstra (Tillie Lewis) *Tasti-Diet*	1 egg	50

Food and Description	Measure or Quantity	Calories
*Scramblers (Morningstar Farms)	1 egg	33
*Second Nature (Avoset)	3 T.	42
ELDERBERRY JELLY (Smucker's)	1 T.	53
ENCHILADA, frozen:		
Beef:		
(Banquet):		
Buffet Supper, with cheese & chili gravy	2-lb. pkg.	1118
Dinner	12-oz. dinner	479
(Green Giant) Sonora style	12-oz. entree	702
(Swanson) *TV Brand*	15-oz. dinner	570
(Van de Kamp's):		
Dinner	12-oz. dinner	390
Entree, shredded	12-oz. entree	420
Cheese:		
(Banquet) *Man-Pleaser*	21¼-oz. dinner	664
(Van de Kamp's)	12-oz. dinner	450
Chicken (Van de Kamp's)	7½-oz. pkg.	250
ENCHILADA SAUCE:		
Canned (Del Monte) hot or mild	½ cup	45
*Mix (Durkee)	½ cup	29
ENDIVE, CURLY OR ESCAROLE, cut up	½ cup	7
ESPRESSO COFFEE LIQUEUR	1 fl. oz.	104

F

FARINA:		
(Hi-O) dry, regular	¼ cup	157
Malt-O-Meal, dry, regular	1 oz.	96
Malt-O-Meal, dry, quick cooking	1 oz.	100
*(Pillsbury) made with milk & salt	⅔ cup	200
FAT, COOKING:		
Crisco:		
Regular	1 T.	110
Butter flavor	1 T.	126
Spry	1 T.	94
FENNEL SEED (French's)	1 tsp.	8
FIG:		
Small	1½″ fig	30
Canned, regular pack (Del Monte) whole, solids & liq.	½ cup	114
Dried, chopped	½ cup	235
FIG JUICE, *RealFig*	½ cup	61
FIGURINES (Pillsbury) all flavors	1 bar	138

Food and Description	Measure or Quantity	Calories
FILBERT:		
Shelled	1 oz.	180
(Fisher) oil dipped, salted	½ cup	360
FISH CAKE, frozen (Mrs. Paul's):		
Breaded & fried	2-oz. cake	105
Thins, breaded & fried	½ of 10-oz. pkg.	326
FISH & CHIPS, frozen:		
(Mrs. Paul's) batter fried, light	½ of 14-oz. pkg.	366
(Swanson):		
Hungry Man	15¾-oz. dinner	820
TV Brand	5-oz. entree	300
(Van de Kamp's) batter dipped, french fried	8-oz. serving	500
FISH DINNER, frozen:		
(Banquet)	8¾-oz. dinner	382
(Mrs. Paul's):		
Au gratin	½ of 10-oz. pkg.	249
Parmesan	½ of 10-oz. pkg.	230
(Van de Kamp's) batter dipped, french fried	11-oz. dinner	540
(Weight Watchers) in lemon sauce, 3-compartment	13¼-oz. meal	250
FISH FILLET, frozen:		
(Mrs. Paul's):		
Batter fried, crunchy	2¼-oz. piece	178
Breaded & fried	2-oz. piece	114
Miniature, batter fried	3-oz. serving	181
(Van de Kamp's):		
Batter dipped, french fried	3-oz. piece	220
Country seasoned	2.4-oz. piece	180
FISH KABOBS, frozen:		
(Mrs. Paul's) light batter	⅓ pkg.	200
(Van de Kamp's):		
Batter dipped	.4-oz. piece	26
Country seasoned	.4-oz. piece	29
FISH SANDWICH, frozen		
(Mrs. Paul's) fillet	4⅛-oz. sandwich	200
FISH SEASONING (Featherweight)	¼ tsp.	<1
FISH STICK, frozen:		
(Mrs. Paul's):		
Batter fried	1 stick	69
Breaded & fried	1 stick	43
(Van de Kamp's) batter dipped, french fried	1-oz. piece	58
FIT 'N FROSTY (Alba '77):		
Chocolate or marshmallow flavor	1 envelope	70
Strawberry	1 envelope	74
Vanilla	1 envelope	69

Food and Description	Measure or Quantity	Calories
FIVE ALIVE (Snow Crop)	6 fl. oz.	85
FLOUNDER:		
Baked	4 oz.	229
Frozen:		
(Mrs. Paul's) fillets, breaded & fried	2-oz. fillet	138
(Mrs. Paul's) with lemon butter	4¼-oz. serving	154
(Weight Watchers) with lemon flavored bread crumbs	6½ oz. serving	134
(Weight Watchers) in Newburgh sauce	12½-oz. pkg.	198
FLOUR:		
(Aunt Jemima) self-rising	¼ cup	109
Ballard, self-rising	¼ cup	100
Bisquick (Betty Crocker)	¼ cup	120
(Elam's):		
Brown rice, whole grain	¼ cup	146
Buckwheat, pure	¼ cup	92
Pastry	1 oz.	102
Rye, whole grain	¼ cup	89
Soy	1 oz.	98
Gold Medal (Betty Crocker) all-purpose or high protein	¼ cup	100
La Pina	¼ cup	100
Pillsbury's Best:		
All-purpose or rye, medium	¼ cup	100
Sauce & gravy	2 T.	50
Self-rising	¼ cup	95
Presto, self-rising	¼ cup	98
Wondra	¼ cup	100
FOOD STICKS (Pillsbury) chocolate	1 stick	45
FRANKEN*BERRY, cereal (General Mills)	1 cup	110
FRANKFURTER:		
(Best's Kosher):		
Regular	1.5-oz. frankfurter	133
Beef	1.5-oz. frankfurter	102
Cocktail	.3-oz. frankfurter	27
Jumbo	2-oz. frankfurter	178
(Eckrich):		
Beef or meat	1.6-oz. frankfurter	150
Beef or meat, jumbo	2-oz. frankfurter	190
Meat	1.2-oz. frankfurter	120
(Hormel):		
Beef	1.6-oz. frankfurter	139
Range Brand, Wrangler, smoked	1 frankfurter	160
(Hygrade) Beef, *Ball Park*	2-oz. franfurter	169

Food and Description	Measure or Quantity	Calories
(Louis Rich) Turkey	1.5-oz. frankfurter	95
(Oscar Mayer):		
Beef	1.6-oz. frankfurter	145
Little Wiener	2" frankfurter	31
Wiener	1.6-oz. frankfurter	145
Wiener, with cheese	1.6-oz. frankfurter	146
(Oscherwitz):		
Regular	1.6-oz. frankfurter	142
Cocktail	.3-oz. frankfurter	27
(Vienna) beef	1.5-oz. frankfurter	132
FRANKS-N-BLANKETS (Durkee)	1 piece	45
FRENCH TOAST, frozen:		
(Aunt Jemima):		
Regular	1½-oz. slice	85
Cinnamon swirl	1 slice	97
(Swanson) with sausage, *TV Brand*	4½-oz. breakfast	270
FRITTERS, frozen (Mrs. Paul's):		
Apple	2-oz. piece	125
Clam	1.9-oz. piece	131
Corn	2-oz. piece	73
Shrimp	½ of 7¾-oz. pkg.	242
FROOT LOOPS, cereal (Kellogg's)	1 cup	110
FROSTED RICE, cereal (Kellogg's)	1 cup	110
FROSTS (Libby's):		
Dry:		
Banana	.5 oz.	50
Orange, strawberry or pineapple	.5 oz.	60
Liquid:		
Banana	7 fl. oz.	120
Orange or strawberry	8 fl. oz.	120
FROZEN DESSERT, dietetic:		
Good Humor:		
Bar, vanilla with chocolate coating	2½-fl. oz. bar	90
Cup, vanilla & chocolate	5-fl. oz. cup	100
(Sugarlo) all flavors	¼ pt.	135
FRUIT COCKTAIL:		
Canned, regular pack, solids & liq.:		
(Del Monte) regular and chunky	½ cup	94
(Libby's)	½ cup	101
(Stokely-Van Camp)	½ cup	95
Canned, dietetic pack, solids & liq.:		
(Del Monte) *Lite*	½ cup	58
(Diet Delight):		
Syrup pack	½ cup	50
Water pack	½ cup	40
(Featherweight):		
Juice pack	½ cup	50
Water pack	½ cup	40

Food and Description	Measure or Quantity	Calories
(Libby's) water pack	½ cup	50
(S&W) *Nutradiet:*		
Juice pack	½ cup	50
Water pack	½ cup	40
***FRUIT COUNTRY** (Comstock):*		
Apple	¼ of pkg.	160
Blueberry	¼ of pkg.	160
Cherry	¼ of pkg.	180
FRUIT CUP (Del Monte):		
Mixed fruits	5-oz. container	110
Peaches, diced	5-oz. container	116
***FRUIT & FIBER,** cereal (Post)*	½ cup	103
FRUIT JUICE, canned (Sun-Maid)	6 fl. oz.	100
FRUIT, MIXED:		
Canned (Del Monte) *Lite,* chunky	½ cup	58
Frozen (Birds Eye) quick thaw	5-oz. serving	150
FRUIT PUNCH:		
Canned:		
Capri Sun	6¾-fl. oz.	102
(Hi-C)	6 fl. oz.	93
(Lincoln) party	6 fl. oz.	100
Chilled:		
Five Alive (Snow Crop)	6 fl. oz.	87
(Minute Maid)	6 fl. oz.	93
*Frozen, *Five Alive* (Snow Crop)	6 fl. oz.	87
*Mix (Hi-C)	6 fl. oz.	72
FRUIT ROLL, frozen (La Choy)	.5-oz. roll	38
***FRUIT ROLL-UPS** (Betty Crocker)*	1 roll	50
FRUIT SALAD:		
Canned, regular pack:		
(Del Monte) fruits for salads	½ cup	93
(Libby's)	½ cup	99
Canned, dietetic pack:		
(Diet Delight)	½ cup	60
(Featherweight):		
Juice pack	½ cup	50
Water pack	½ cup	40
(S&W) *Nutradiet:*		
Juice pack	½ cup	60
Water pack	½ cup	35
***FRUIT SQUARES,** frozen*		
(Pepperidge Farm)	2½-oz. piece	230
***FUDGSICLE** (Popsicle Industries)*	2½-fl.-oz. bar	100

Food and Description	Measure or Quantity	Calories

G

GARLIC:
Flakes (Gilroy)	1 tsp.	5
Powder (French's)	1 tsp.	5
Spread (Lawry's)	1 T.	79

GEFILTE FISH, canned:
(Mother's):
Jelled, old world	4-oz. serving	70
Jelled, whitefish & pike	4-oz. serving	60
In liquid broth	4-oz. serving	70

(Rokeach):
Jelled, Whitefish & Pike	4-oz. serving	50
Old Vienna	4-oz. serving	70

GELATIN, dry, *Caramel Kosher*	7-gram envelope	30

*GELATIN DESSERT MIX:
Regular:
Carmel Kosher, all flavors	½ cup	80
(Jell-O) all flavors	½ cup	81

Dietetic:
Carmel Kosher	½ cup	8
(D-Zerta) all flavors	½ cup	6
(Estee) all flavors	½ cup	40
(Featherweight) artificially sweetened or regular	½ cup	10

GELATIN, DRINKING (Knox) range	1 envelope	70

GERMAN STYLE DINNER
(Swanson) *TV Brand*	11¾-oz. dinner	370

GIN, SLOE:
(Bols)	1 fl. oz.	85
(DeKuyper)	1 fl. oz.	70
(Hiram Walker)	1 fl. oz.	68
(Mr. Boston)	1 fl. oz.	68

GIN & TONIC, canned (Party Tyme)
10% alcohol	2 fl. oz.	55

GINGER, powder (French's)	1 tsp.	6

*GINGERBREAD MIX:
(Betty Crocker)	⅑ of cake	210
(Dromedary)	2″ × 2″ square	100
(Pillsbury)	3″ square	190

GOLDEN GRAHAMS, cereal
(General Mills)	¾ cup	110
GOOBER GRAPE (Smucker's)	1 oz.	125

GOOD HUMOR (See ICE CREAM)

Food and Description	Measure or Quantity	Calories
GOOD N' PUDDIN (Popsicle Industries) all flavors	2¼-fl.-oz. bar	170
GOOSE, roasted, meat & skin	4 oz.	500
GRAHAM CRAKOS, cereal (Kellogg's)	1 cup	110
GRANOLA BARS, *Nature Valley:*		
Almond, cinnamon or oats 'n honey	1 bar	110
Coconut or peanut	1 bar	120
*GRANOLA BAR MIX, chewy (Nature Valley) *Bake-A-Bar*	1 bar	100
GRANOLA CEREAL:		
Nature Valley:		
Cinnamon & raisin, fruit & nut or toasted oat	⅓ cup	130
Coconut & honey	⅓ cup	150
Sun Country:		
With almonds	½ cup	253
With raisins	½ cup	241
GRANOLA CLUSTERS, *Nature Valley:*		
Almond	1 roll	140
Caramel & raisin	1 roll	150
GRANOLA & FRUIT BAR, *Nature Valley*	1 bar	150
GRANOLA SNACK, *Nature Valley*	1 pouch	140
GRAPE:		
American rype (slipskin)	3½″ × 3″ bunch	43
Canned, dietetic (Featherweight) light, seedless, water pack	½ cup	60
GRAPE DRINK:		
Canned:		
Capri Sun	1¾ fl. oz.	104
(Hi-C)	6 fl. oz.	89
(Lincoln)	6 fl. oz.	96
(Welchade)	6 fl. oz.	90
*Frozen (Welchade)	6 fl. oz.	90
*Mix (Hi-C)	6 fl. oz.	68
GRAPEFRUIT:		
Pink & red:		
Seeded type	½ med. grapefruit	46
Seedless type	½ med. grapefruit	49
White:		
Seeded type	½ med. grapefruit	44
Seedless type	½ med. grapefruit	46
Canned, regular pack (Del Monte) in syrup	½ cup	74
Canned, dietetic pack, solids & liq.: (Del Monte) sections	½ cup	45

Food and Description	Measure or Quantity	Calories
(Diet Delight) sections	½ cup	45
(Featherweight) sections, juice pack	½ cup	40
(S&W) *Nutradiet,* sections	½ cup	40
GRAPEFRUIT DRINK, canned		
(Lincoln)	6 fl. oz.	104
GRAPEFRUIT JUICE:		
Fresh, pink, red or white	½ cup	46
Canned, sweetened:		
(Del Monte)	6 fl. oz.	89
(Texsun)	6 fl. oz.	77
Canned, unsweetened:		
(Del Monte)	6 fl. oz.	72
(Ocean Spray)	6 fl. oz.	64
(Texsun)	6 fl. oz.	77
Chilled (Minute Maid)	6 fl. oz.	75
GRAPEFRUIT JUICE COCKTAIL, canned (Ocean Spray) pink	6 fl. oz.	84
GRAPEFRUIT-ORANGE JUICE COCKTAIL, canned, *Musselman's*	6 fl. oz.	67
GRAPE JAM (Smucker's)	1 T.	53
GRAPE JELLY:		
Sweetened:		
(Smucker's)	1 T.	53
(Welch's)	1 T.	52
Dietetic (See GRAPE SPREAD)		
GRAPE JUICE:		
Canned, unsweetened:		
(Seneca Foods)	6 fl. oz.	118
(Welch's)	6 fl. oz.	120
*Frozen:		
(Minute Maid)	6 fl. oz.	99
(Welch's)	6 fl. oz.	100
GRAPE JUICE DRINK, chilled		
(Welch's)	6 fl. oz.	110
GRAPE NUTS, cereal (Post):		
Regular	¼ cup	108
Flakes	⅞ cup	108
GRAPE SPREAD, dietetic:		
(Diet Delight)	1 T.	12
(Estee)	1 T.	18
(Featherweight) calorie reduced	1 T.	16
(Smucker's)	1 T.	24
(Welch's)	1 T.	30
GRAVY, canned:		
Au jus (Franco-American)	2-oz. serving	10
Beef (Franco-American)	2-oz. serving	25

Food and Description	Measure or Quantity	Calories
Brown:		
(Franco-American) with onion	2-oz. serving	25
(La Choy)	5-oz. can	417
Ready Gravy	¼ cup	44
Chicken:		
(Franco-American)	2-oz. serving	50
(Franco-American) giblet	2-oz. serving	30
Mushroom (Franco-American)	2-oz. serving	25
Turkey (Franco-American)	2-oz. serving	30
GRAVYMASTER	1 tsp.	11
GRAVY WITH MEAT OR TURKEY:		
Canned (Morton House):		
Sliced beef	6¼-oz. serving	190
Sliced turkey	6¼-oz. serving	140
Frozen:		
(Banquet):		
Giblet gravy & sliced turkey, *Cookin' Bag*	5-oz. bag	98
Sliced beef, *Buffet Supper*	2-lb. pkg.	782
(Swanson) sliced beef with whipped potatoes, *TV Brand*	8-oz. entree	200
GRAVY MIX:		
Regular:		
Au jus:		
*(Durkee)	½ cup	15
*(French's) *Gravy Makins*	½ cup	16
Brown:		
*(Durkee):		
Regular	½ cup	29
With mushrooms	½ cup	29
*(French's) *Gravy Makins*	½ cup	40
*(Pillsbury)	½ cup	30
*(Spatini)	1-oz. serving	8
Chicken:		
(Durkee):		
*Regular	½ cup	43
Roastin' Bag	1½-oz. pkg.	122
*(French's) *Gravy Makins*	½ cup	50
*(Pillsbury)	½ cup	50
Home style:		
*(Durkee)	½ cup	35
*(French's) *Gravy Makins*	½ cup	50
*(Pillsbury)	½ cup	30
Meatloaf (Durkee) *Roastin' Bag*	1½-oz. pkg.	129
Mushroom:		
*(Durkee)	½ cup	30
*(French's) *Gravy Makins*	½ cup	40

Food and Description	Measure or Quantity	Calories
Onion:		
*(Durkee)	½ cup	42
*(French's) *Gravy Makins*	½ cup	50
Pork:		
*(Durkee)	½ cup	35
*(French's) *Gravy Makins*	½ cup	40
*Swiss steak (Durkee)	½ cup	23
Turkey:		
*(Durkee)	½ cup	47
*(French's) *Gravy Makins*	½ cup	50
*Dietetic (Weight Watchers):		
Brown	½ cup	16
Brown, with mushrooms	½ cup	24
Brown, with onion	½ cup	26
Chicken	½ cup	20
GREENS, MIXED, canned		
(Sunshine) solids & liq.	½ cup	20
GRENADINE (Garnier) no alcohol	1 fl. oz.	103
GUAVA	1 guava	48
GUAVA NECTAR (Libby's)	6 fl. oz.	70

H

HADDOCK:		
Fried, breaded	4″ × 3″ × ½″ fillet	165
Frozen:		
(Banquet)	8¾-oz. dinner	419
(Mrs. Paul's) breaded & fried	2-oz. fillet	114
(Swanson) filet almondine	7½-oz. entree	370
(Van de Kamp's) batter dipped, french fried	2-oz. piece	165
(Weight Watchers) with stuffing, 2-compartment	7-oz. pkg.	205
Smoked	4-oz. serving	117
HALIBUT:		
Broiled	4″ × 3″ × ½″ steak	214
Frozen (Van de Kamp's) batter dipped, french fried	½ of 8-oz. pkg.	270
HAM:		
Canned:		
(Hormel):		
Chunk	6¾-oz. serving	329
Chopped	¼ of 12-oz. can	229
Patties	1 patty	200

Food and Description	Measure or Quantity	Calories
(Oscar Mayer) *Jubilee*, extra lean, cooked	1-oz. serving	31
(Swift):		
Hostess	3½-oz. slice	141
Premium	1¾-oz. slice	111
Deviled:		
(Libby's)	1 oz.	87
(Underwood)	1 oz.	98
Packaged:		
(Eckrich) cooked, sliced	1.2-oz. slice	37
(Hormel):		
Black or red peppered	.8-oz. slice	26
Chopped	1-oz. slice	61
Cooked	.8-oz. slice	26
(Oscar Mayer):		
Chopped	1-oz. slice	64
Cooked, smoked	¾-oz. slice	25
Cooked, smoked	1-oz. slice	34
Jubilee, sliced, boneless	8-oz. slice	264
Jubilee, steak, boneless, 95% fat free	2-oz. steak	69
HAMBURGER (See *McDONALD'S, BURGER KING, DAIRY QUEEN, WHITE CASTLE*, etc.)		
HAMBURGER MIX:		
Hamburger Helper (General Mills):		
Beef noodle	⅕ of pkg.	320
Cheeseburger	⅕ of pkg.	360
Hash	⅕ of pkg.	300
Lasagna	⅕ of pkg.	330
Pizza	⅕ of pkg.	320
Potatoes au gratin	⅕ of pkg.	320
Rice oriental	⅕ of pkg.	320
Stew	⅕ of pkg.	290
Make a Better Burger (Lipton) mildly seasoned or onion	⅕ of pkg.	30
HAMBURGER SEASONING MIX:		
*(Durkee)	1 cup	663
(French's)	1-oz. pkg.	100
HAM & CHEESE:		
(Hormel) loaf	1-oz. serving	69
(Oscar Mayer) loaf	1-oz. serving	77
HAM DINNER, frozen:		
(Banquet)	10-oz. dinner	369
(Swanson) *TV Brand*	10¼-oz. dinner	320
HAM SALAD, canned (Carnation)	1½-oz. serving	84
HAM SALAD SPREAD		
(Oscar Mayer)	1 oz.	62

Food and Description	Measure or Quantity	Calories
HAWAIIAN PUNCH:		
Canned:		
Cherry	6 fl. oz.	87
Grape	6 fl. oz.	93
Red	6 fl. oz.	84
Very berry	6 fl. oz.	87
*Mix, red punch	8 fl. oz.	100
HEADCHEESE (Oscar Mayer)	1-oz. serving	54
HERRING, canned (Vita):		
Cocktail, drained	8-oz. jar	342
In cream sauce	8-oz. jar	397
Tastee Bits, drained	8-oz. jar	361
HERRING, SMOKED, kippered	4-oz. serving	239
HICKORY NUT, shelled	1-oz. serving	191
HO-HO (Hostess)	1-oz. cake	126
HOMINY GRITS:		
Dry:		
(Albers)	1½ oz.	150
(Aunt Jemima)	3 T.	102
(Quaker):		
Regular	3 T.	101
Instant:		
Regular	.8-oz. packet	79
With imitation bacon or ham	1-oz. packet	101
Cooked	1 cup	125
HONEY, strained	1 T.	61
HONEYCOMB, cereal (Post)	1⅓ cups	112
HONEYDEW	2″ × 7″ wedge	31
HORSERADISH:		
Raw, pared	1 oz.	25
Prepared (Gold's)	1-oz. serving	18
HOSTESS O's (Hostess)	2¼-oz. piece	277

I

ICE CREAM (listed by type, such as sandwich or *Whammy*, or by flavor); (See also FROZEN DESSERT):		
Bar (Good Humor) vanilla, chocolate coated	3-fl.-oz. piece	170
Bar (Heath) *Butter Brickle,* chocolate coated	2½-fl.-oz. piece	154
Butter pecan:		
(Breyer's)	¼ pt.	180
(Good Humor) bulk	4 fl. oz.	150
Cherry, black (Good Humor) bulk	4 fl. oz.	130

Food and Description	Measure or Quantity	Calories
Chocolate:		
(Baskin-Robbins):		
Regular	1 scoop (2½ fl. oz.)	165
Fudge	1 scoop (2½ fl. oz.)	178
(Good Humor) bulk	4 fl. oz.	130
(Swift's) sweet cream	2¼ fl. oz. (½ cup)	129
Chocolate chip (Good Humor)	4 fl. oz.	150
Chocolate chip cookie		
(Good Humor)	1 sandwich	480
Chocolate eclair, bar (Good Humor)	3-fl.-oz. piece	220
Coffee (Breyer's)	¼ pt.	140
Eskimo Pie, vanilla with chocolate		
coating	3-fl.-oz. bar	180
Eskimo Thin Mint, with chocolate		
coating	2-fl.-oz. bar	140
Fudge royal (Good Humor) bulk	4 fl. oz.	120
Peach (Breyer's)	¼ pt.	130
Pralines 'N Cream (Baskin-Robbins)	1 scoop (2½ fl. oz.)	177
Sandwich (Good Humor)	2½-oz. piece	200
Strawberry:		
(Baskin-Robbins)	1 scoop (2½ fl. oz.)	141
(Good Humor) bulk	4 fl. oz.	120
Strawberry shortcake (Good Humor)	3-fl.-oz. piece	200
Toasted almond bar (Good Humor)	3-fl.-oz. piece	220
Toffee fudge swirl (Good Humor)		
bulk	4 fl. oz.	130
Vanilla:		
(Baskin-Robbins) regular	1 scoop (2½ oz.)	147
(Good Humor) bulk	4 fl. oz.	140
(Swift's) sweet cream	½ cup	127
Vanilla-chocolate-strawberry (Good		
Humor) bulk	4 fl. oz.	130
Vanilla fudge swirl (Good Humor)		
bulk	4 fl. oz.	140
Whammy (Good Humor):		
Assorted	1.6-oz. piece	100
Chip crunch bar	1.6-oz. piece	110
ICE CREAM CONE, cone only		
(Comet):		
Regular	1 piece	20
Rolled sugar	1 piece	40
ICE CREAM CUP, cup only (Comet)	1 cup	20
***ICE CREAM MIX** (Salada) any		
flavor	1 cup	310
ICE MILK:		
Hardened	¼ pt.	100

Food and Description	Measure or Quantity	Calories
Soft-serve	¼ pt.	133
(Dean) *Count Calorie*	¼ pt.	99
(Meadow Gold) vanilla, 4% fat	¼ pt.	95
ITALIAN DINNER, frozen (Banquet)	11-oz. dinner	446

J

Food and Description	Measure or Quantity	Calories
JELLO PUDDING POPS:		
Banana, butterscotch or vanilla	2-oz. pop	96
Chocolate or chocolate fudge	2-oz. pop	101
JELLY, sweetened (See also individual flavors) (Crosse & Blackwell) all flavors	1 T.	51
JERUSALEM ARTICHOKE, pared	4 oz.	75
JOHANNISBERG RIESLING:		
(Deinhard)	3 fl. oz.	72
(Inglenook)	3 fl. oz.	61

K

Food and Description	Measure or Quantity	Calories
KABOOM, cereal (General Mills)	1 cup	110
KALE:		
Boiled, leaves only	4 oz.	44
Canned (Sunshine) chopped, solids & liq.	½ cup	21
Frozen:		
(Birds Eye) chopped	⅓ of pkg.	32
(McKenzie) chopped	3⅓ oz.	25
(Southland) chopped	⅕ of 16-oz. pkg.	30
KARO SYRUP (See SYRUP)		
KEFIR (Alta-Dena Dairy):		
Plain	1 cup	180
Flavored	1 cup	190
KIDNEY:		
Beef, braised	4 oz.	286
Calf, raw	4 oz.	128
Lamb, raw	4 oz.	119
KIELBASA:		
(Eckrich) skinless	2-oz. serving	190
(Hormel) Kolbase	2-oz. serving	245
(Vienna)	2-oz. serving	165
KING VITAMAN, cereal (Quaker)	1¼ cups	113

Food and Description	Measure or Quantity	Calories
KIRSCH, liqueur (Garnier)	1 fl. oz.	83
KIX, cereal	1½ cups	110
KNOCKWURST (Best's Kosher; Oscherwitz):		
Regular	3-oz. piece	270
Beef	3-oz. piece	203
KOOL-AID (General Foods):		
Unsweetened (sugar to be added)	8 fl. oz.	93
Pre-sweetened:		
All flavors except tropical punch	8 fl. oz.	93
Tropical punch	8 fl. oz.	98
KUMQUAT, flesh & skin	5 oz.	74

L

LAMB:		
Leg:		
Roasted, lean & fat	3 oz.	237
Roasted, lean only	3 oz.	158
Loin, one 5-oz. chop (weighed with bone before cooking) will give you:		
Lean & fat	2.8 oz.	280
Lean only	2.3 oz.	122
Rib, one 5-oz. chop (weighed with bone before cooking) will give you:		
Lean & fat	2.9 oz.	334
Lean only	2 oz.	118
Shoulder:		
Roasted, lean & fat	3 oz.	287
Roasted, lean only	3 oz.	174
LASAGNA:		
Canned:		
(Hormel) *Short Orders*	7½-oz. can	260
(Nalley's)	8-oz. serving	239
Frozen:		
(Green Giant):		
Bake:		
Regular, with meat *sauce*	12-oz. entree	465
Chicken	12-oz. entree	640
Boil 'N Bag	9-oz. entree	311
(Swanson):		
Regular, with meat in tomato sauce	13¼-oz. entree	480
Hungry Man, with meat	17¾-oz. dinner	690
TV BRAND	13-oz. dinner	420

Food and Description	Measure or Quantity	Calories
(Weight Watchers)	12¾-oz. meal	409
LEEKS	4 oz.	59
LEMON:		
Whole	2⅛" lemon	22
Peeled	2⅛" lemon	20
LEMONADE:		
Canned:		
Capri Sun	6¾ fl. oz.	63
Country Time	6 fl. oz.	69
(Hi-C)	6 fl. oz.	68
Chilled (Minute Maid) regular or pink	6 fl. oz.	79
*Frozen:		
Country Time, regular or pink	6 fl. oz.	68
Minute Maid	6 fl. oz.	74
*Mix:		
Country Time, regular or pink	6 fl. oz.	68
(Hi-C)	6 fl. oz.	76
Kool Aid, sweetened, regular or pink	6 fl. oz.	75
Lemon Tree (Lipton)	6 fl. oz.	68
(Minute Maid) regular or pink	6 fl oz.	80
LEMON EXTRACT (Virginia Dare)	1 tsp.	21
LEMON JUICE:		
Canned, *ReaLemon*	1 T.	3
*Frozen (Minute Maid) unsweetened	1 fl. oz.	7
***LEMON-LIMEADE**, mix (Minute Maid)	6 fl. oz.	80
LEMON PEEL, candied	1 oz.	90
LEMON-PEPPER SEASONING (French's)	1 tsp.	6
LENTIL, cooked, drained	½ cup	107
LETTUCE:		
Bibb or Boston	4" head	23
Cos or Romaine, shredded or broken into pieces	½ cup	4
Grand Rapids, Salad Bowl or Simpson	2 large leaves	9
Iceberg, New York or Great Lakes	¼ of 4¾" head	15
LIEBFRAUMILCH WINE (Deinhard)	3 fl. oz.	60
LIFE, cereal (Quaker) regular or cinnamon	⅔ cup	105
LIL' ANGELS (Hostess)	1-oz. piece	78
LIME, peeled	2" dia.	15
***LIMEADE,** frozen (Minute Maid)	6 fl. oz.	75
LIME JUICE, *ReaLime*	1 T.	2

Food and Description	Measure or Quantity	Calories
LIVER:		
Beef:		
Fried	6½″ × 2⅜″ × ⅜″ slice	195
Cooked (Swift)	3.2-oz. serving	141
Calf, fried	6½″ × 2⅜″ × ⅜″ slice	222
Chicken, simmered	2″ × 2″ × ⅝″ liver	41
LIVERWURST SPREAD		
(Underwood)	1-oz. serving	92
LOBSTER:		
Cooked, meat only	1 cup	138
Canned, meat only	4-oz. serving	108
Frozen, South African lobster tail:		
3 in 8-oz. pkg.	1 piece	87
4 in 8-oz. pkg.	1 piece	65
5 in 8-oz. pkg.	1 piece	51
LOBSTER NEWBURG	1 cup	485
LOBSTER PASTE, canned	1-oz. serving	51
LOBSTER SALAD	4-oz. serving	125
LOG CABIN SYRUP (See SYRUP)		
LONG ISLAND TEA COCKTAIL,		
canned (Mr. Boston)	3 fl. oz.	92
LOQUAT, fresh, flesh only	2 oz.	27
LUCKY CHARMS, cereal (General		
Mills)	1 cup	110
LUNCHEON MEAT (See also		
individual listings, e.g., BOLOGNA,		
HAM, etc.)		
All meat (Oscar Mayer)	1-oz. slice	98
Bar-B-Que loaf (Oscar Mayer) 90%		
fat free	1-oz. slice	49
Beef honey roll sausage (Oscar		
Mayer) 90% fat free	.8-oz. slice	40
Beef, jellied (Hormel) loaf	1.2-oz. slice	35
Ham & cheese (See HAM &		
CHEESE)		
Ham roll sausage (Oscar Mayer)	.8-oz. slice	35
Ham roll sausage (Oscar Mayer)	1-oz. slice	43
Honey loaf:		
(Eckrich)	1-oz. slice	40
(Hormel)	1-oz. slice	47
Honey loaf (Oscar Mayer) 95% fat		
free	1-oz. slice	37
Liver cheese (Oscar Mayer)	1.3-oz. slice	114
Liver loaf (Hormel)	1-oz. slice	81
Luxury loaf (Oscar Mayer) 95% fat		
free	1-oz. slice	39
Meat loaf	1-oz. serving	57

Food and Description	Measure or Quantity	Calories
New England brand sliced sausage:		
(Hormel)	1-oz. slice	49
(Oscar Mayer) 92% fat free	.5-oz. slice	22
(Oscar Mayer) 92% fat free	.8-oz. slice	34
Old fashioned loaf (Oscar Mayer)	1-oz. slice	65
Olive loaf:		
(Hormel)	1-oz. slice	59
(Oscar Mayer)	1-oz. slice	65
Peppered loaf:		
(Hormel)	1-oz. serving	72
(Oscar Mayer) 93% fat free	1-oz. slice	42
Pickle loaf:		
(Eckrich)	1-oz. slice	85
(Hormel)	1-oz. slice	59
Pickle & pimiento (Oscar Mayer)	1-oz. slice	65
Picnic loaf (Oscar Mayer)	1-oz. slice	64
Spiced (Hormel)	1-oz. serving	77

M

Food and Description	Measure or Quantity	Calories
MACADAMIA NUT		
(Royal Hawaiian)	1 oz.	197
MACARONI:		
Cooked:		
8-10 minutes, firm	1 cup	192
14-20 minutes, tender	1 cup	155
Canned:		
(Franco-American):		
Beefy Mac	7½-oz. can	220
PizzOs	7½-oz. can	170
(Nalley's) & beef	8 oz.	236
Frozen:		
(Banquet) & beef:		
Regular	12-oz. dinner	394
Buffet Supper	2-lb. pkg.	1000
(Swanson) *TV Brand*, & beef	12-oz. dinner	370
MACARONI & CHEESE;		
Canned:		
(Franco-American) regular or elbow	7⅜-oz. serving	170
(Hormel) *Short Orders*	7½-oz. can	170
Frozen:		
(Banquet):		
Buffet Supper	2-lb. pkg.	1027
Dinner	12-oz. dinner	326

Food and Description	Measure or Quantity	Calories
(Green Giant), Boil 'N Bag	9-oz. entree	286
(Swanson):		
Regular	12-oz. entree	440
TV Brand	12¼-oz. dinner	380
Mix:		
(Golden Grain) deluxe	¼ of 7¼-oz. pkg.	202
*(Lipton)	¼ of pkg.	210
*(Prince)	¾ cup	268
MACARONI & CHEESE PIE, frozen		
(Swanson)	7-oz. pie	210
MACARONI SALAD, canned		
(Nalley's)	4-oz. serving	206
MACKEREL, Atlantic, broiled, with		
fat	8½″ × 2½″ × ½″ fillet	248
MADEIRA WINE (Leacock)	3 fl. oz.	120
MAI TAI COCKTAIL:		
Canned:		
(National Distillers) *Duet,* 12½%		
alcohol	8-fl.-oz. can	288
(Party Tyme) 12½% alcohol	2 fl. oz.	65
Mix:		
Dry (Bar-Tender's; Holland		
House)	1 serving	69
Liquid, canned (Holland House)	1½ fl. oz.	50
MALTED MILK MIX (Carnation):		
Chocolate	3 heaping tsps.	85
Natural	3 heaping tsps.	88
MALT LIQUOR, *Champale,* regular	12 fl. oz.	179
MALT-O-MEAL, cereal	1 T.	33
MANDARIN ORANGE (See		
TANGERINE)		
MANGO, fresh	1 med. mango	88
MANGO NECTAR (Libby's)	6 fl. oz.	60
MANHATTAN COCKTAIL:		
Canned (Mr. Boston) 20% alcohol	3 fl. oz.	123
Mix, dry (Bar-Tender's)	1 serving	24
Mix, liquid, canned (Holland House)	1½ fl. oz.	14
MAPLE SYRUP (See SYRUP, Maple)		
MARGARINE:		
Regular	1 pat (1″ × 1.3″ × 1″,	
	5 grams)	36
(Mazola)	1 T.	104
(Parkay) regular, soft or squeeze	1 T.	101
MARGARINE, IMITATION OR		
DIETETIC:		
(Parkay)	1 T.	55
(Weight Watchers)	1 T.	50

Food and Description	Measure or Quantity	Calories
MARGARINE, WHIPPED (Blue Bonnet; Miracle; Parkay)	1 T.	67
MARGARITA COCKTAIL:		
Canned (Mr. Boston):		
Regular, 12½% alcohol	3 fl. oz.	105
Strawberry, 12½% alcohol	3 fl. oz.	138
Mix:		
Dry (Bar-Tender's)	1 serving	70
Liquid (Holland House)	1½ fl. oz.	58
MARINADE MIX:		
Chicken (Adolph's)	1-oz. packet	64
Meat:		
(Adolph's)	.8-oz. pkg.	38
(Durkee)	1-oz. pkg.	47
(French's)	1-oz. pkg.	80
MARJORAM (French's)	1 tsp.	4
MARMALADE:		
Sweetened:		
(Keiller)	1 T.	60
(Smucker's)	1 T.	53
Dietetic:		
(Dia-Mel)	1 T.	6
(Featherweight)	1 T.	16
(Smucker's) imitation	1 T.	24
(S&W) *Nutradiet*	1 T.	12
MARSHMALLOW FLUFF	1 heaping tsp.	59
MARSHMALLOW KRISPIES, cereal (Kellogg's)	1¼ cups	140
MARTINI COCKTAIL:		
Gin, canned (Mr. Boston) extra dry, 20% alcohol	3 fl. oz.	99
Gin, mix, liquid (Holland House)	2 fl. oz.	20
Vodka, canned (Mr. Boston) 20% alcohol	3 fl. oz.	108
MASA HARINA (Quaker)	⅓ cup	137
MASA TRIGO (Quaker)	⅓ cup	149
MATZO (Horowitz Margareten) regular	1 matzo	120
MAYONNAISE:		
Real, *Hellmann's* (Best Foods)	1 T.	103
Imitation or dietetic:		
(Diet Delight) *Mayo-Lite*	1 T.	24
(Featherweight) *Soyamaise*	1 T.	100
(Tillie Lewis) *Tasti-Diet*, *Maylonaise*	1 T.	25
(Weight Watchers)	1 T.	40
MAYPO, cereal:		
30-second	¼ cup	89

Food and Description	Measure or Quantity	Calories
Vermont-style	¼ cup	121
McDONALD'S:		
Big Mac	1 hamburger	563
Biscuit:		
Ham	1 piece	422
Sausage	1 piece	582
Cheeseburger	1 hamburger	307
Chicken McNuggets	1 serving	314
Cookies:		
Chocolate Chip	1 package	342
McDonaldland	1 package	308
Egg McMuffin	1 serving	327
Egg, scrambled	1 serving	180
English muffin, with butter	1 muffin	186
Filet-O-Fish	1 sandwich	432
Grapefruit juice	6 fl. oz.	80
Hamburger	1 hamburger	255
Hot cakes with butter & syrup	1 serving	500
McChicken Sandwich	1 sandwich	475
McFeast	1 serving	485
McRib	1 sandwich	455
Orange juice	6 fl. oz.	85
Pie:		
Apple	1 pie	253
Cherry	1 pie	260
Potato:		
Fried	1 regular order	220
Hash browns	1 order	125
Quarter Pounder	1 hamburger	424
Quarter Pounder with cheese	1 hamburger	524
Sausage, pork	1 serving	206
Shake:		
Chocolate	1 serving	383
Strawberry	1 serving	362
Vanilla	1 serving	352
Sundae:		
Caramel	1 sundae	328
Hot Fudge	1 sundae	310
Strawberry	1 sundae	289
MEATBALL DINNER or ENTREE,		
frozen:		
(Green Giant)	9.9-oz. entree	371
(Swanson) *TV Brand*	9¼-oz. entree	320
MEATBALL SEASONING MIX:		
*(Durkee) Italian style	1 cup	619
(French's)	1½-oz. pkg.	140
MEATBALL STEW, canned:		
Dinty Moore	7½-oz. serving	245

Food and Description	Measure or Quantity	Calories
(Libby's)	12-oz. serving	281
(Nalley's)	8-oz. serving	261
MEATBALLS, SWEDISH, frozen		
(Stouffer's) with noodles	11-oz. pkg.	473
MEAT LOAF DINNER, frozen:		
(Banquet):		
Regular	11-oz. dinner	412
Man-Pleaser	19-oz. dinner	916
(Swanson):		
TV Brand	10¾-oz. dinner	490
TV Brand, with tomato sauce and whipped potatoes	9-oz. entree	340
MEAT LOAF SEASONING MIX (French's)	1½-oz. pkg.	160
MEAT, POTTED (Libby's)	1-oz. serving	55
MEAT SEASONING, dietetic (Featherweight)	¼ tsp.	<1
MEAT TENDERIZER (Adolph's)	1 tsp.	2
MELBA TOAST, salted (Old London):		
Garlic, onion or white rounds	1 piece	10
Pumpernickel, rye, wheat or white	1 piece	17
Sesame, flat	1 piece	18
MELON BALL, in syrup, frozen	½ cup	72
MEXICAN DINNER, frozen:		
(Banquet) combination	12-oz. dinner	571
(Swanson) *TV Brand*	16-oz. dinner	590
(Van de Kamp's) combination	11-oz. dinner	430
MILK, CONDENSED, *Dime Brand; Eagle Brand; Magnolia Brand*	1 T.	60
*MILK, DRY, non-fat, instant (Alba; Carnation; Pet; *Sanalac*)	1 cup	80
MILK, EVAPORATED:		
Regular:		
(Carnation)	1 fl. oz.	42
(Pet)	1 fl. oz.	43
Filled:		
Dairymate	½ cup	150
(Pet)	½ cup	150
Low Fat (Carnation)	1 fl. oz.	27
Skimmed:		
(Carnation)	1 fl. oz.	25
Pet 99	1 fl. oz.	25
MILK, FRESH:		
Buttermilk (Friendship)	8 fl. oz.	120
Chocolate (Dairylea)	8 fl. oz.	180
Low Fat, *Viva,* 2% fat	8 fl. oz.	130
Skim (Dairylea; Meadow Gold)	1 cup	90

Food and Description	Measure or Quantity	Calories
Whole:		
(Dairylea)	1 cup	150
(Meadow Gold)	1 cup	120
MILK, GOAT, whole	1 cup	163
MILK, HUMAN	1 oz.	22
MILNOT, dairy vegetable blend	1 fl. oz.	38
MINERAL WATER (Schweppes)	6 fl. oz.	0
MINI-WHEATS, cereal	1 biscuit	28
MINT LEAVES	½ oz.	4
MOLASSES:		
Barbados	1 T.	51
Blackstrap	1 T.	40
Dark (Brer Rabbit)	1 T.	33
Light	1 T.	48
Medium	1 T.	44
Unsulphured (Grandma's)	1 T.	60
MORTADELLA sausage	1 oz.	89
MOSELLE WINE (Great Western)	3 fl. oz.	72
MOST, cereal (Kellogg's)	½ cup	100
MOUSSE, canned, dietetic (Featherweight) chocolate	½ cup	100
MUFFIN:		
Blueberry:		
(Hostess)	1¾-oz. muffin	127
(Pepperidge Farm) regular or frozen	1.9-oz. muffin	180
Bran (Arnold) *Bran'nola*	2.3-oz. muffin	160
Corn:		
(Pepperidge Farm)	1.9-oz. muffin	180
(Thomas')	2-oz. muffin	184
English:		
(Arnold) extra crisp	2.3-oz. muffin	150
(Pepperidge Farm):		
Plain	2-oz. muffin	130
Cinnamon apple	2-oz. muffin	140
Wheat	2-oz. muffin	130
Roman Meal	2⅓-oz. muffin	150
(Thomas') regular or frozen	2-oz. muffin	133
(Wonder)	2-oz. muffin	133
Orange-Cranberry (Pepperidge Farm)	2.1-oz. muffin	190
Plain	1.4-oz. muffin	118
Raisin (Arnold)	2.5-oz. muffin	170
Sourdough (Wonder)	2-oz. muffin	131
MUFFIN MIX:		
Blueberry:		
*(Betty Crocker) wild	1 muffin	120
(Duncan Hines)	1/12 of pkg.	99

Food and Description	Measure or Quantity	Calories
Bran (Duncan Hines)	1/12 of pkg.	97
*Cherry (Betty Crocker)	1/12 of pkg.	120
Corn:		
*(Betty Crocker)	1 muffin	160
*(Dromedary)	1 muffin	130
*(Flako)	1 muffin	140
MULLIGAN STEW, canned, *Dinty Moore, Short Orders*	7½-oz. can	230
MUSCATEL WINE (Gallo) 14% alcohol	3 fl. oz.	86
MUSHROOM:		
Raw, whole	½ lb.	62
Raw, trimmed, sliced	½ cup	10
Canned:		
(Green Giant)	2-oz. serving	14
(Shady Oaks)	4-oz. can	19
Frozen (Green Giant) whole, in butter sauce	3-oz. serving	42
MUSHROOM, CHINESE, dried	1 oz.	81
MUSHROOM SOUP (See SOUP, Mushroom)		
MUSSEL, in shell	1 lb.	153
MUSTARD:		
Powder (French's)	1 tsp.	9
Prepared:		
Brown (French's; Gulden's; *Grey Poupon*)	1 tsp.	5
Dijon, *Grey Poupon*	1 tsp.	6
Horseradish (Nalley's)	1 tsp.	5
Unsalted (Featherweight)	1 tsp.	5
Yellow (Gulden's)	1 tsp.	5
MUSTARD GREENS:		
Canned (Sunshine) solids & liq.	½ cup	22
Frozen:		
(Birds Eye)	1/3 of pkg.	25
(McKenzie)	1/3 of pkg.	20
(Seabrook Farms)	1/3 of pkg.	25
(Southland)	1/3 of 16-oz. pkg.	20
MUSTARD SPINACH:		
Raw	1 lb.	100
Boiled, drained, no added salt	4-oz. serving	18

N

NATURAL CEREAL:
  Heartland:

Regular	¼ cup	120
Coconut	¼ cup	130
(Quaker):		
Hot, whole wheat	⅓ cup	106
100%	¼ cup	138
100% with apple & cinnamon	¼ cup	135
100% with raisins & dates	¼ cup	134
NATURE SNACKS (Sun-Maid):		
Carob Crunch	1 oz.	143
Raisin Crunch	1 oz.	126
Rocky Road	1 oz.	126
Tahitian Treat	1 oz.	123
Yogurt Crunch	1 oz.	123
NECTARINE, flesh only	4 oz.	73
NOODLE:		
Dry (Pennsylvania Dutch Brand)		
broad	1 oz.	105
Cooked, 1½″ strips	1 cup	200
NOODLES & BEEF:		
Canned (Hormel) *Short Orders*	7½-oz. can	230
Frozen (Banquet) *Buffet Supper*	2-lb. pkg.	754
NOODLE & CHICKEN:		
Canned, *Dinty Moore, Short Orders*	7½-oz. can	210
Frozen (Swanson) *TV Brand*	10½-oz. dinner	270
NOODLE, CHOW MEIN:		
(Chun King)	⅙ of 5-oz. can	100
(La Choy)	½ cup	149
NOODLE MIX:		
(Betty Crocker):		
Fettucine Alfredo	¼ of pkg.	220
Romanoff	¼ of pkg.	230
Stroganoff	¼ of pkg.	240
Noodle Roni, parmesano	⅕ of 6-oz. pkg.	130
(Lipton) Egg Noodles & Sauce:		
Beef, butter or chicken	¼ pkg.	190
Butter & Herb	¼ pkg.	180
Cheese	¼ pkg.	200
***NOODLE, RAMEN** (La Choy)*		
canned:		
Beef	½ of 3-oz. can	189

Food and Description	Measure or Quantity	Calories
Chicken	½ of 3-oz. can	187
Oriental	½ of 3-oz. can	190
NOODLE, RICE (La Choy)	1 oz.	130
NOODLE ROMANOFF, frozen		
(Stouffer's)	⅓ of pkg.	168
NUT, MIXED:		
Dry roasted:		
(A&P)	1 oz.	179
(Flavor House)	1 oz.	172
(Planters)	1 oz.	160
Oil roasted:		
(Excel) with peanuts	1 oz.	187
(Planters) with peanuts	1 oz.	180
(Planters) without peanuts	1 oz.	180
NUTMEG (French's)	1 tsp.	11
NUT*Os (General Mills)	1 T.	35
NUTRI-GRAIN, cereal (Kellogg's):		
Corn	½ cup	110
Wheat	⅔ cup	110
NUTRIMATO (Mott's)	6 fl. oz.	70

O

Food and Description	Measure or Quantity	Calories
OAT FLAKES, cereal (Post)	⅔ cup	107
OATMEAL:		
Dry:		
Regular:		
(Elam's) Scotch style	1 oz.	108
(H-O) old fashioned	1 T.	15
(Quaker) old fashioned	⅓ cup	109
(Ralston Purina)	⅓ cup	110
Instant:		
(H-O):		
Regular, boxed	1 T.	15
Regular, packets	1-oz. packet	105
With bran & spice	1½-oz. packet	157
With cinnamon & spice	1⅝-oz. packet	175
With maple & brown sugar flavor	1½-oz. packet	160
(Quaker):		
Regular	1-oz. packet	105
Apple & cinnamon	1¼-oz. packet	134
Bran & raisin	1½-oz. packet	153
Maple & brown sugar	1½-oz. packet	163
Raisins & spice	1½-oz. packet	159

Food and Description	Measure or Quantity	Calories
(3-Minute Brand) *Stir'N Eat:*		
Dutch apple brown sugar	1⅛-oz. packet	120
Natural flavor	1-oz. packet	106
Quick:		
(Harvest Brand)	⅓ cup	108
(H-O)	½ cup	129
(Quaker) old fashioned	⅓ cup	109
(Ralston Purina)	⅓ cup	110
(3-Minute Brand)	⅓ cup	108
Cooked, regular	1 cup	132
OIL, SALAD or COOKING:		
Crisco; Fleischmann's; Mazola; Puritan	1 T.	126
Golden Thistle; Mrs. Tucker's; Planters	1 T.	130
Saffola	1 T.	124
Sunlite; Wesson	1 T.	120
OKRA, frozen:		
(Birds Eye) whole	⅓ of pkg.	36
(McKenzie) cut	⅓ of pkg.	25
(Seabrook Farms) cut	⅓ of pkg.	32
(Seabrook Farms) whole	⅓ of pkg.	36
(Southland) cut	⅕ of 16-oz. pkg.	25
OLD FASHIONED COCKTAIL:		
Canned (Hiram Walker) 62 proof	3 fl. oz.	165
Mix, dry (Bar-Tender's)	1 serving	20
OLIVE:		
Green	4 med. or 3 extra large or 2 giant	19
Ripe, Mission	3 small or 2 large	18
OMELET, frozen (Swanson) *TV Brand*, Spanish style	7¾-oz. entree	240
ONION:		
Raw	2½″ onion	38
Boiled, pearl onion	½ cup	27
Canned (Durkee) *O & C:*		
Boiled	¼ of 16-oz. jar	32
Creamed	¼ of 15½-oz. can	554
Dehydrated (Gilroy) flakes	1 tsp.	5
Frozen:		
(Birds Eye):		
Chopped	1 oz.	9
Creamed	⅓ of pkg.	106
Whole	⅓ of pkg.	44
(Green Giant) cheese sauce	⅓ of pkg.	63
(Mrs. Paul's) french-fried rings	½ of 5-oz. pkg.	157
(Southland) chopped	⅕ of 10-oz. pkg.	20

Food and Description	Measure or Quantity	Calories
ONION BOUILLON:		
(Croydon House)	1 tsp.	11
(Herb-Ox)	1 cube	10
MBT	1 packet	16
ONION, GREEN	1 small onion	4
ONION SALAD SEASONING		
(French's) instant	1 T.	15
ONION SALT (French's)	1 tsp.	6
ONION SOUP (See SOUP, onion)		
*ON*YOS* (General Mills)	1 T.	35
ORANGE:		
Peeled	½ cup	62
Sections	4 oz.	58
ORANGE-APRICOT JUICE		
COCKTAIL, *Musselman's*	8 fl. oz.	100
ORANGE DRINK:		
Canned:		
Capri Sun	6¾-oz. can	103
(Hi-C)	8 fl. oz.	123
(Lincoln)	8 fl. oz.	128
*Mix (Hi-C)	8 fl. oz.	91
ORANGE EXTRACT:		
(Durkee) imitation	1 tsp.	14
(Virginia Dare)	1 tsp.	22
ORANGE-GRAPEFRUIT JUICE:		
Canned (Del Monte):		
Sweetened	6 fl. oz.	91
Unsweetened	6 fl. oz.	79
*Frozen (Minute Maid) unsweetened	6 fl. oz.	76
ORANGE JUICE:		
Canned:		
(Del Monte) sweetened	6 fl. oz.	76
(Libby's) unsweetened	6 fl. oz.	90
(Sunkist) unsweetened	½ cup	60
(Texsun) sweetened	6 fl. oz.	83
Chilled (Minute Maid)	6 fl. oz.	83
*Frozen:		
Bright & Early, imitation	6 fl. oz.	90
(Minute Maid) unsweetened	6 fl. oz.	86
(Snow Crop)	6 fl. oz.	86
(Sunkist)	6 fl. oz.	92
ORANGE PEEL, candied	1 oz.	93
ORANGE-PINEAPPLE DRINK,		
canned (Lincoln)	8 fl. oz.	128
ORANGE-PINEAPPLE JUICE,		
canned (Texsun)	6 fl. oz.	89
ORANGE-PINEAPPLE JUICE		
COCKTAIL, *Musselman's*	8 fl. oz.	100

Food and Description	Measure or Quantity	Calories
*ORANGE PLUS (Birds Eye)	6 fl. oz.	98
ORANGE SPREAD, dietetic (Estee)	1 tsp.	8
OVALTINE, chocolate	¾ oz.	78
OVEN FRY (General Foods):		
Crispy crumb for pork	4.2-oz. envelope	484
Extra crispy for chicken	4.2-oz. envelope	462
Traditional pork	5.3-oz. envelope	539
OYSTER:		
Raw:		
Eastern	19-31 small or 13-19 med.	158
Pacific & Western	6-9 small or 4-6 med.	218
Canned (Bumble) shelled, whole, solids & liq.	1 cup	218
Fried	4 oz.	271
OYSTER STEW, home recipe	½ cup	103

P

*PAC-MAN CEREAL (General Mills)	1 cup	110
*PANCAKE BATTER, FROZEN (Aunt Jemima):		
Plain	4" pancake	70
Blueberry or buttermilk	4" pancake	68
PANCAKE & SAUSAGE, frozen (Swanson)	6-oz. entree	440
*PANCAKE & WAFFLE MIX:		
Plain:		
(Aunt Jemima):		
Complete	4" pancake	80
Original	4" pancake	73
(Log Cabin):		
Complete	4" pancake	58
Original	4" pancake	60
(Pillsbury) Hungry Jack:		
Complete, bulk or packets	4" pancake	60
Extra Lights	4" pancake	67
Golden Blend, complete	4" pancake	80
Panshakes	4" pancake	83
Blueberry (Pillsbury) Hungry Jack	4" pancake	107
Buckwheat (Aunt Jemima)	4" pancake	67
Buttermilk:		
(Aunt Jemima):		
Regular	4" pancake	100
Complete	4" pancake	80

Food and Description	Measure or Quantity	Calories
(Betty Crocker):		
Regular	4" pancake	93
Complete	4" pancake	70
(Pillsbury) *Hungry Jack*, complete	4" pancake	63
Whole wheat (Aunt Jemima)	4" pancake	83
Dietetic:		
(Featherweight)	4" pancake	43
(Tillie Lewis) *Tasti-Diet*	4" pancake	47
PANCAKE & WAFFLE SYRUP		
(See SYRUP, Pancake & Waffle)		
PAPAYA, fresh:		
Cubed	½ cup	36
Juice	4 oz.	78
PAPRIKA (French's)	1 tsp.	7
PARSLEY:		
Fresh, chopped	1 T.	2
Dried (French's)	1 tsp.	4
PASSION FRUIT, giant, whole	1 lb.	53
PASTINAS, egg	1 oz.	109
PASTRAMI:		
(Eckrich) sliced	1-oz. serving	47
(Vienna)	1-oz. serving	86
PASTRY SHEET, PUFF, frozen (Pepperidge Farm)	4.3-oz. sheet	510
PASTRY SHELL, frozen (Pepperidge Farm)	1 patty shell	210
PÂTÉ:		
De foie gras	1 T.	69
Liver (Hormel)	1 T.	35
PDQ:		
Chocolate	1 T.	66
Strawberry	1 T.	60
PEA, green:		
Boiled	½ cup	58
Canned, regular pack, solids & liq.:		
(Del Monte):		
Early	½ cup	55
Seasoned	½ cup	54
(Festal) sweet, tiny	½ cup	50
(Green Giant):		
Early, with onions	½ cup	62
Sweet	½ cup	49
Sweet, with onion	½ cup	62
(Libby's) sweet	½ cup	66
(Stokely-Van Camp) early	½ cup	65
Canned, dietetic pack, solids & liq.:		
(Diet Delight)	½ cup	50
(Featherweight) sweet	½ cup	70

Food and Description	Measure or Quantity	Calories
(S&W) *Nutradiet*, sweet	½ cup	40
Frozen:		
(Birds Eye):		
Regular	⅓ of pkg. (3.3 oz.)	78
In cream sauce	⅓ of pkg. (2.7 oz.)	84
With sliced mushrooms	⅓ of pkg.	75
(Green Giant):		
Creamed	⅓ of pkg.	83
Early & sweet in butter sauce	3⅓ oz.	75
Sweet, *Harvest Fresh*	4 oz.	85
(McKenzie) regular	⅓ of pkg.	80
(Seabrook Farms)	⅓ of pkg.	77
PEA & CARROT:		
Canned, regular pack, solids & liq.:		
(Del Monte)	½ cup	49
(Libby's)	½ cup	56
Canned, dietetic pack, solids & liq.:		
(Diet Delight)	½ cup	40
(S&W) *Nutradiet*	½ cup	35
Frozen:		
(Bird's Eye)	3.3 oz.	61
(McKenzie)	3.3 oz.	60
PEA, CHOWDER, frozen (Southland)	⅕ of 16-oz. pkg.	120
PEA POD:		
Boiled, drained solids	4 oz.	49
Frozen (La Choy)	6-oz. pkg.	90
PEACH:		
Fresh, with thin skin	2″ peach	38
Fresh, slices	½ cup	32
Canned, regular pack, solids & liq.:		
(Del Monte):		
Cling	4 oz.	95
Spiced	7¼ oz.	170
(Libby's):		
Halves, heavy syrup	½ cup	105
Sliced, heavy syrup	½ cup	102
Canned, dietetic pack, solids & liq.:		
(Del Monte) Lite, Cling	½ cup	53
(Diet Delight):		
Cling, syrup pack	½ cup	50
Cling, water pack	½ cup	30
(Featherweight):		
Cling or Freestone, juice pack	½ cup	50
Cling, water pack	½ cup	30
(Libby's) water pack, Lite	½ cup	50
(S&W) *Nutradiet:*		
Cling, juice pack	½ cup	60
Cling, water pack	½ cup	30

Food and Description	Measure or Quantity	Calories
Freestone, juice pack	½ cup	50
Frozen (Birds Eye)	5 oz.	141
PEACH BUTTER (Smucker's)	1 T.	45
PEACH DRINK (Hi-C):		
Canned	6 fl. oz.	90
*Mix	6 fl. oz.	72
PEACH LIQUEUR (DeKuyper)	1 fl. oz.	82
PEACH NECTAR (Libby's)	6 fl. oz.	90
PEACH PRESERVE OR JAM:		
Sweetened (Smucker's)	1 T.	53
Dietetic:		
(Dia-Mel)	1 T.	6
(Featherweight)	1 T.	16
(Featherweight) artificially sweetened	1 T.	6
PEACH SPREAD, dietetic (Tillie Lewis) *Tasti-Diet*	1 T	12
PEANUT:		
Dry roasted:		
(Fisher)	1 oz.	163
(Frito-Lay)	1 oz.	173
(Planters)	1 oz.	160
Oil roasted (Planters)	1 oz. (jar)	179
PEANUT BUTTER:		
Regular:		
(Elam's) natural with defatted wheat germ	1 T.	109
(Jif) creamy	1 T.	93
(Peter Pan):		
Crunchy	1 T.	101
Smooth	1 T.	94
(Planters) crunchy or smooth	1 T.	95
(Skippy):		
Creamy	1 T.	108
Creamy, old fashioned	1 T.	107
(Smucker's):		
Creamy or crunchy	1 T.	90
Natural	1 T.	100
Dietetic:		
(Featherweight) low sodium	1 T.	90
(Peter Pan) low sodium	1 T.	106
(S&W) *Nutradiet*, low sodium	1 T.	93
PEANUT BUTTER BAKING CHIPS (Reese's)	3 T. (1 oz.)	151
PEAR:		
Whole	3″ × 2½″ pear	101
Canned, regular pack, solids & liq.:		
(Del Monte) Bartlett	½ cup	88

Food and Description	Measure or Quantity	Calories
(Libby's)	½ cup	94
Canned, dietetic pack, solids & liq.:		
(Del Monte) *Lite*	½ cup	57
(Featherweight):		
Bartlett, juice pack	½ cup	60
Bartlett, water pack	½ cup	40
(Libby's) water pack	½ cup	60
(S&W) *Nutradiet:*		
Juice pack	½ cup	60
Water pack	½ cup	35
Dried (Sun-Maid)	½ cup	260
PEAR NECTAR (Libby's)	6 fl. oz.	100
PEAR-PASSION FRUIT NECTAR		
(Libby's)	6 fl. oz.	60
PEBBLES, cereal:		
Cocoa	⅞ cup	117
Fruity	⅞ cup	116
PECAN:		
Halves	6–7 pieces	48
Roasted, dry:		
(Fisher) salted	1 oz.	220
(Planters)	1 oz.	190
PECTIN, FRUIT:		
Certo	6 oz.	19
Sure-Jell	1¾-oz. pkg.	170
PEP, cereal (Kellogg's)	¾ cup	110
PEPPER:		
Black (French's)	1 tsp.	9
Lemon (Durkee)	1 tsp.	1
Seasoned (French's)	1 tsp.	8
PEPPER, CHILI, canned:		
(Del Monte):		
Green, whole	½ cup	20
Jalapeno or chili, whole	½ cup	30
Old El Paso, green, chopped or		
whole	1 oz.	7
(Ortega):		
Diced, strips or whole	1 oz.	6
Jalapeno, diced or whole	1 oz.	9
PEPPERMINT EXTRACT (Durkee)		
imitation	1 tsp.	15
PEPPERONI:		
(Hormel) sliced	1-oz. serving	142
(Swift)	1-oz. serving	152
PEPPER & ONION, frozen		
(Southland):		
Diced	2 oz.	15
Red & green	2 oz.	20

Food and Description	Measure or Quantity	Calories
PEPPER STEAK, frozen:		
*(Chun King) stir fry	⅕ of pkg.	70
(Stouffer's)	5¼-oz. serving	354
PEPPER, STUFFED:		
Home recipe	2¾" × 2½" pepper with 1⅛ cups stuffing	314
Frozen:		
(Green Giant) green, baked	7 oz.	219
(Weight Watchers) with veal stuffing	11¾ oz.	238
PEPPER, SWEET:		
Raw:		
Green:		
Whole	1 lb.	82
Without stem & seeds	1 med. pepper (2.6 oz.)	13
Red:		
Whole	1 lb.	112
Without stem & seeds	1 med. pepper (2.2 oz.)	19
Boiled, green, without salt, drained	1 med. pepper (2.6 oz.)	13
Frozen:		
(McKenzie) green	1 oz.	6
(Southland):		
Green	2 oz.	10
Red & green	2 oz.	15
PERCH, OCEAN:		
Atlantic, raw:		
Whole	1 lb.	124
Meat only	4 oz.	108
Pacific, raw, whole	1 lb.	116
Frozen:		
(Banquet)	8¾-oz. dinner	434
(Mrs. Paul's) fillet, breaded & fried	2-oz. piece	127
(Van de Kamp's)	2-oz. piece	145
(Weight Watchers)	6½-oz. meal	160
PERNOD (Julius Wile)	1 fl. oz.	79
PERSIMMON:		
Japanese or Kaki, fresh:		
With seeds	4.4-oz. piece	79
Seedless	4.4-oz. piece	81
Native, fresh, flesh only	4 oz.	144
PHEASANT, raw, meat only	4 oz.	184

Food and Description	*Measure or Quantity*	*Calories*
PICKLE:		
Cucumber, fresh or bread & butter:		
(Fannings)	1.2-oz.	17
(Featherweight)	1-oz. pickle	12
(Nalley's) chips	1 oz.	27
Dill:		
(Featherweight) whole, low sodium	1 oz.	4
(Nalley's) regular & Polish style	1 oz.	3
(Smucker's):		
Hamburger, sliced	1 slice	<1
Polish, whole	3½" pickle	8
Spears	3½" spear	6
Hamburger (Nalley's) chips	1 oz.	3
Kosher dill:		
(Claussen) halves or whole	2 oz.	7
(Featherweight) low sodium	1 oz.	4
(Smucker's):		
Baby	2¾" long pickle	4
Slices	1 slice	<1
Whole	2½" long pickle	8
Sweet:		
(Nalley's):		
Regular	1 oz.	37
Nubbins	1 oz.	28
(Smucker's):		
Candied mix	1 piece	14
Gherkins	2" long pickle	15
Whole	2½" long pickle	18
Sweet & sour (Claussen) slices	1 slice	3
PIE:		
Regular:		
Apple:		
Home recipe, two-crust	⅙ of 9" pie	404
(Hostess)	4½-oz. pie	409
Banana, home recipe, cream or custard	⅙ of 9" pie	336
Berry (Hostess)	4½-oz. pie	404
Blackberry, home recipe, two-crust	⅙ of 9" pie	384
Blueberry:		
Home recipe, two-crust	⅙ of 9" pie	382
(Hostess)	4½-oz. pie	394
Boston cream, home recipe	1/12 of 8" pie	208
Butterscotch, home recipe, one-crust	⅙ of 9" pie	406
Cherry:		
Home recipe, two-crust	⅙ of 9" pie	412
(Hostess)	4½-oz. pie	429

Food and Description	Measure or Quantity	Calories
Chocolate chiffon, home recipe	1/6 of 9" pie	459
Chocolate meringue, home recipe	1/6 of 9" pie	353
Coconut custard, home recipe	1/6 of 9" pie	357
Lemon (Hostess)	4½-oz. pie	415
Mince, home recipe, two-crust	1/6 of 9" pie	428
Peach (Hostess)	4½-oz. pie	409
Pecan (Frito-Lay)	3-oz. serving	353
Pumpkin, home recipe, one-crust	1/6 of 9" pie	321
Raisin, home recipe, two-crust	1/6 of 9" pie	427
Rhubarb, home recipe, two-crust	1/6 of 9" pie	400
Strawberry (Hostess)	4½-oz. pie	367
Frozen:		
Apple:		
(Banquet)	1/5 of 20-oz. pie	288
(Morton):		
Regular	1/6 of 24-oz. pie	295
Great Little Desserts	8-oz. pie	598
(Sara Lee):		
Regular	1/6 of 31-oz. pie	376
Dutch	1/6 of 30-oz. pie	354
Banana cream:		
(Banquet)	1/6 of 14-oz. pie	172
(Morton):		
Regular	1/6 of 16-oz. pie	174
Great Little Desserts	3½-oz. pie	237
Blueberry:		
(Banquet)	1/6 of 20-oz. pie	253
(Morton):		
Regular	1/6 of 24-oz. pie	286
Great Little Desserts	8-oz. pie	589
(Sara Lee)	1/6 of 31-oz. pie	449
Cherry:		
(Banquet)	1/6 of 20-oz. pie	228
(Morton):		
Regular	1/6 of 24-oz. pie	300
Great Little Desserts	8-oz. pie	589
(Sara Lee)	1/6 of 31-oz. pie	397
Chocolate cream:		
(Banquet)	1/6 of 14-oz. pie	177
(Morton) regular	1/6 of 16-oz. pie	199
Coconut cream:		
(Banquet)	1/6 of 14-oz. pie	179
(Morton):		
Regular	1/6 of 16-oz. pie	197
Great Little Desserts	2½-oz. pie	266
Coconut custard:		
(Banquet)	1/6 of 20-oz. pie	203
(Morton) *Great Little Desserts*	6½-oz. pie	369

Food and Description	Measure or Quantity	Calories
Custard (Banquet)	⅕ of 20-oz. pie	247
Lemon cream:		
(Banquet)	⅙ of 14-oz. pie	168
(Morton):		
Regular	⅙ of 16-oz. pie	182
Great Little Desserts	3½-oz. pie	245
Mince:		
(Banquet)	⅙ of 20-oz. pie	252
(Morton)	⅙ of 24-oz. pie	314
Peach:		
(Banquet)	⅕ of 20-oz. pie	263
(Sara Lee)	⅙ of 31-oz. pie	458
Pumpkin:		
(Banquet)	⅙ of 20-oz. pie	206
(Morton)	⅙ of 24-oz. pie	235
(Sara Lee)	⅛ of 45-oz. pie	354
Strawberry cream:		
(Banquet)	⅙ of 14-oz. pie	169
(Morton)	⅙ of 16-oz. pie	182
PIECRUST:		
Home recipe, 9″ pie	1 crust	900
Frozen (Banquet) 9″ pie shell:		
Regular	1 crust	614
Deep dish	1 crust	751
*PIECRUST MIX:		
(Betty Crocker) regular or stick:		
Regular	¹⁄₁₆ pkg.	120
Stick	⅛ stick	120
(Flako)	⅙ of 9″ pie shell	245
(Pillsbury) mix or stick	⅙ of 2-crust shell	270
PIE FILLING (See also PUDDING OR PIE FILLING):		
Apple (Comstock)	⅙ of 21-oz. can	110
Apple rings or slices (See APPLE, canned)		
Apricot (Comstock)	⅙ of 21-oz. can	110
Banana cream (Comstock)	⅙ of 21-oz. can	110
Blueberry (Comstock)	⅙ of 21-oz. can	120
Cherry (Comstock)	⅙ of 21-oz. can	120
Coconut cream (Comstock)	⅙ of 21-oz. can	120
Coconut custard, home recipe, made with egg yolk & milk	5 oz. (inc. crust)	288
Lemon (Comstock)	⅙ of 21-oz. can	160
Mincemeat (Comstock)	⅙ of 21-oz. can	170
Peach (Comstock)	⅙ of 21-oz. can	130
Pineapple (Comstock)	⅙ of 21-oz. can	110
Pumpkin (Libby's) (See also PUMPKIN, canned)	1 cup	210

Food and Description	Measure or Quantity	Calories
Raisin (Comstock)	⅙ of 21-oz. can	140
Strawberry (Comstock)	⅙ of 21-oz. can	130
*PIE MIX (Betty Crocker) Boston cream	⅛ of pie	260
PIEROGIES, frozen (Mrs. Paul's):		
Cabbage	5-oz. serving	333
Potato & cheese	5-oz. serving	304
Sauerkraut, Polish-style	5-oz. serving	312
PIGS FEET, pickled	4 oz.	226
PIMIENTO, canned:		
(Dromedary)	1-oz. serving	10
(Ortega)	¼ cup	6
(Sunshine) diced or sliced	1 T.	4
PINA COLADA:		
Canned (Mr. Boston) 12½% alcohol	3 fl. oz.	240
Mix:		
Dry (Party Tyme)	½-oz. pkg.	50
Liquid (Holland House)	2 fl. oz.	120
PINEAPPLE:		
Fresh, chunks	½ cup	52
Canned, regular pack, solids & liq.:		
(Del Monte) slices, medium	½ cup	92
(Dole):		
Chunk, crushed or sliced, juice pack	½ cup	70
Chunk, crushed or sliced, heavy syrup	½ cup	95
Canned, unsweetened or dietetic, solids & liq.:		
(Del Monte):		
Chunks, juice pack	½ cup	70
Crushed, juice pack	½ cup	77
Slices, juice pack	½ cup	81
(Diet Delight) juice pack	½ cup	70
(Featherweight):		
Juice pack	½ cup	70
Water pack	½ cup	60
(Libby's) Lite	½ cup	60
(S&W) Nutradiet, slices	1 slice	30
PINEAPPLE, CANDIED	1 oz.	90
PINEAPPLE FLAVORING (Durkee) imitation	1 tsp.	6
PINEAPPLE & GRAPEFRUIT JUICE DRINK, canned:		
(Del Monte) regular or pink	6 fl. oz.	98
(Dole) pink	6 fl. oz.	101
(Texsun)	6 fl. oz.	91

Food and Description	Measure or Quantity	Calories
PINEAPPLE JUICE:		
Canned:		
(Del Monte) with vitamin C	6 fl. oz.	108
(Dole)	6 fl. oz.	103
(Texsun)	6 fl. oz.	97
*Frozen (Minute Maid)	6 fl. oz.	92
PINEAPPLE-ORANGE DRINK,		
canned (Hi-C)	6 fl. oz.	94
PINEAPPLE-ORANGE JUICE:		
Canned (Del Monte)	6 fl. oz.	97
*Frozen (Minute Maid)	6 fl. oz.	94
PINEAPPLE PRESERVE OR JAM,		
sweetened (Smucker's)	1 T.	53
PINE NUT, pignolias, shelled	1 oz.	156
PINOT CHARDONNAY WINE		
(Paul Masson) 12% alcohol	3 fl. oz.	71
PISTACHIO NUT:		
In shell	½ cup	197
Shelled	¼ cup	184
(Fisher) shelled, roasted, salted	1 oz.	174
PIZZA PIE:		
Regular, non-frozen:		
Home recipe	⅛ of 14″ pie	177
(Pizza Hut):		
Cheese	½ of 10″ pie	436
Pepperoni	½ of 10″ pie	459
Pork	½ of 10″ pie	475
Frozen:		
Canadian style bacon (Celeste)	8-oz. pie	483
Cheese:		
(Celeste)	½ of 7-oz. pie	236
(Celeste)	¼ of 19-oz. pie	309
(Stouffer's) French bread	½ of 10¼-oz. pkg.	330
Totino's	½ of pie	440
(Weight Watchers)	6-oz. pie	364
Combination:		
(Celeste) Chicago style	¼ of 24-oz. pie	360
(La Pizzeria)	½ of 13½-oz. pie	420
Totino's, classic	⅓ of pie	520
(Van de Kamp's) thick crust	¼ of 23.5-oz. pie	310
(Weight Watchers) deluxe	7¼-oz. pie	322
Deluxe:		
(Celeste)	½ of 9-oz. pie	281
(Celeste)	¼ of 23½-oz. pie	368
(Stouffer's) French bread	½ of 12⅜-oz. pkg.	400
Hamburger (Stouffer's) French bread	½ of 12¼-oz. pkg.	397
Mexican style (Van de Kamp's)	½ of 11-oz. pie	420

Food and Description	Measure or Quantity	Calories
Pepperoni:		
(Celeste)	½ of 7¼-oz. pie	284
(Celeste)	¼ of 20-oz. pie	347
(Stouffer's) French bread	½ of 11½oz. pkg.	410
Totino's	½ of pie	460
(Van de Kamp's) thick crust	¼ of 22-oz. pie	370
Sausage:		
(Celeste)	½ of 8-oz. pie	262
(Celeste)	¼ of 22-oz. pie	359
(Stouffer's) French bread	½ of 12-oz. pkg.	420
Totino's	½ of pie	470
Totino's, deep crust	⅙ of pie	300
(Weight Watchers)	6¾-oz. pie	350
Sausage & mushroom:		
(Celeste)	½ of 9-oz. pie	277
(Celeste)	¼ of 24-oz. pie	365
(Stouffer's) French bread	½ of 12½-oz. pkg.	395
Sicilian style (Celeste) deluxe	¼ of 26-oz. pie	408
Suprema (Celeste):		
Regular	½ of 10-oz. pie	295
Without meat	½ of 8-oz. pie	217
Vegetable (Weight Watchers)	7¼-oz. pie	396
PIZZA PIE MIX:		
Regular (Jeno's)	½ of pkg.	420
Cheese:		
(Jeno's)	½ of pkg.	420
(Ragú) Pizza Quick	⅛ of 12″ pie	140
Skillet Pizza (General Mills)	¼ of pkg.	210
Pepperoni:		
(Jeno's)	½ of pkg.	510
Skillet Pizza (General Mills)	¼ of pkg.	220
Sausage, *Skillet Pizza* (General Mills)	¼ of pkg.	230
PIZZA SAUCE:		
(Contadina):		
Regular or with pepperoni	½ cup	80
With cheese	½ cup	90
(Ragu) regular or *Pizza Quick*	5-oz. serving	120
PIZZA SEASONING SPICE		
(French's)	1 tsp.	4
PLUM:		
Fresh, Japanese & hybrid	2″ plum	27
Fresh, prune-type, halves	½ cup	60
Canned, regular pack (Stokely-Van Camp)	½ cup	120
Canned, purple, unsweetened or dietetic, solids & liq.:		
(Diet Delight) juice pack	½ cup	70

Food and Description	Measure or Quantity	Calories
(Featherweight):		
Juice pack	½ cup	80
Water pack	½ cup	40
(S&W) *Nutradiet,* juice pack	½ cup	80
PLUM JELLY (Featherweight)	1 T.	16
PLUM PRESERVE OR JAM,		
Sweetened (Smucker's)	1 T.	53
P.M. FRUIT DRINK (Mott's)	6 fl. oz.	90
POLYNESIAN-STYLE DINNER,		
frozen (Swanson) *TV Brand*	12-oz. dinner	350
POMEGRANATE, whole	1 lb.	160
PONDEROSA RESTAURANT:		
A-1 sauce	1 tsp.	4
Beef, chopped (patty only):		
Regular	3½ oz.	209
Big	4.8 oz.	295
Double Deluxe	5.9 oz.	362
Junior (*Square Shooter*)	1.6 oz.	98
Steakhouse Deluxe	2.96 oz.	181
Beverages:		
Coca-Cola	8 fl. oz.	96
Coffee	6 fl. oz.	2
Dr. Pepper	8 fl. oz.	96
Milk:		
Regular	8 fl. oz.	159
Chocolate	8 fl. oz.	208
Orange drink	8 fl. oz.	110
Root beer	8 fl. oz.	104
Sprite	8 fl. oz.	95
Tab	8 fl. oz.	1
Tea	6 fl. oz.	2
Bun:		
Regular	2.4-oz. bun	190
Hot dog	1 bun	108
Junior	1.4-oz. bun	118
Steakhouse Deluxe	2.4-oz. bun	190
Butter	1 pat (1 tsp.)	36
Catsup	1 T.	18
Chicken strips:		
Adult	2¾ oz.	282
Child	1.4 oz.	141
Cocktail sauce	1½ oz.	57
Filet Mignon	3.8 oz. (edible portion)	152
Filet of Sole, fish only (see also Bun)	3-oz. piece	125
Fish, baked	4.9-oz. serving	268
Gelatin dessert	½ cup	97
Gravy, Au Jus	1 oz.	3

Food and Description	Measure or Quantity	Calories
Ham & cheese:		
Bun (see Bun)		
Cheese, Swiss	2 slices (.8 oz.)	76
Ham	2½ oz.	184
Hot dog, child's, meat only (see also Bun)	1.6-oz. hot dog	140
Lemon wedge		5
Lettuce (see Salad Bar)		
Margarine:		
Pat	1 tsp.	36
On potato, as served	½ oz.	100
Mayonnaise	1 T.	101
Mustard	1 T.	12
Mustard sauce, sweet & sour	1 oz.	50
New York strip steak	6.1 oz. (edible portion)	362
Onion, chopped	1 T. (.4 oz.)	4
Pickle, dill	3 slices (.7 oz.)	2
Potato:		
Baked	7.2 oz.	145
French fries	3 oz.	230
Prime Rib:		
Regular	4.2 oz. (edible portion)	286
Imperial	8.4 oz. (edible portion)	572
King	6 oz. (edible portion)	409
Pudding:		
Butterscotch	4½ oz.	200
Chocolate	4½ oz.	213
Vanilla	4½ oz.	195
Ribeye	3.2 oz. (edible portion)	197
Ribeye & Shrimp:		
Ribeye	3.2 oz.	197
Shrimp	2.2 oz.	139
Roll, kaiser	2.2-oz. roll	184
Salad bar:		
Bean sprouts	1 oz.	13
Beets	1 oz.	5
Broccoli	1 oz.	9
Cabbage, red	1 oz.	9
Carrots	1 oz.	12
Cauliflower	1 oz.	8
Celery	1 oz.	4
Chickpeas (Garbanzos)	1 oz.	102
Cucumber	1 oz.	4
Lettuce	1 oz.	4

Food and Description	Measure or Quantity	Calories
Mushrooms	1 oz.	8
Onions, white	1 oz.	11
Pepper, green	1 oz.	6
Radish	1 oz.	5
Tomato	1 oz.	6
Salad dressing:		
Blue cheese	1 oz.	129
Italian, creamy	1 oz.	138
Low calorie	1 oz.	14
Oil & vinegar	1 oz.	124
Sweet'n tart	1 oz.	129
Thousand island	1 oz.	117
Shrimp dinner	7 pieces (3½ oz.)	220
Sirloin:		
Regular	3.3 oz. (edible portion)	220
Super	6½ oz. (edible portion)	383
Tips	4 oz. (edible portion)	192
Steak sauce	1 oz.	23
Tartar sauce	1½ oz.	285
T-Bone	4.3 oz. (edible portion)	240
Tomato (see also Salad bar):		
Slices	2 slices (.9 oz.)	5
Whole, small	3.5 oz.	22
Topping, whipped	¼ oz.	19
Worcestershire sauce	1 tsp.	4
POPCORN:		
*Plain, popped:		
(Jiffy Pop)	½ of 5-oz. pkg.	244
(Pillsbury) Microwave Popcorn:		
Regular	1 cup	70
Butter flavor	1 cup	65
Packaged:		
Buttered (Old London)	1 cup	57
Caramel-coated:		
(Bachman)	1-oz. serving	130
(Old London):		
Without peanuts	1¾-oz. bag	195
With peanuts	1 cup	142
Cheese flavored (Bachman)	1-oz. serving	180
Cracker Jack	¾-oz. serving	90
*POPOVER MIX (Flako)	1 popover	170
POPPY SEED (French's)	1 tsp.	13
POPSICLE, twin pop	3-fl.-oz. pop	70

Food and Description	Measure or Quantity	Calories
POP TARTS (See TOASTER CAKE OR PASTRY)		
PORK:		
Fresh:		
Chop:		
Broiled, lean & fat	3-oz. chop (weighed without bone)	332
Broiled, lean only	3-oz. chop (weighed without bone)	230
Loin:		
Roasted, lean & fat	3 oz.	308
Roasted, lean only	3 oz.	216
Spareribs, braised	3 oz.	374
Cured ham:		
Roasted, lean & fat	3 oz.	246
Roasted, lean only	3 oz.	159
PORK DINNER (Swanson)		
TV Brand	11¼-oz. dinner	270
PORK RINDS, *Baken-Ets*	1-oz. serving	150
PORK STEAK, BREADED, frozen (Hormel)	3-oz. serving	223
PORK, SWEET & SOUR, frozen:		
(Chun King)	½ of 15-oz. pkg.	220
(La.Choy)	½ of 15-oz. pkg.	229
PORT WINE:		
(Gallo)	3 fl. oz.	94
(Great Western)	3 fl. oz.	138
(Louis M. Martini)	6 fl. oz.	165
POSTUM, instant	6 fl. oz.	11
POTATO:		
Cooked:		
Au gratin	½ cup	127
Baked, peeled	2½″ dia. potato	92
Boiled, peeled	4.2-oz. potato	79
French-fried	10 pieces	156
Hash-browned, home recipe	½ cup	223
Mashed, milk & butter added	½ cup	92
Canned:		
(Del Monte) drained	8 oz.	130
(Sunshine) whole, solids & liq.	1 cup	102
Frozen:		
(Birds Eye):		
Cottage fries	2.8-oz. serving	119
Crinkle cuts, regular	3-oz. serving	115
French fries, regular	3-oz. serving	113
Hash browns, shredded	¼ of 12-oz. pkg.	61
Tasti Puffs	¼ of 10-oz. pkg.	192
Tiny Taters	⅓ of 16-oz. pkg.	204

Food and Description	Measure or Quantity	Calories
Whole, peeled	3.2 oz.	59
(Green Giant):		
Sliced, in butter sauce	3.3 oz.	44
& sweet peas in bacon cream		
sauce	3.3 oz.	97
(McKenzie) whole, white	3.2 oz.	60
(Seabrook Farms) whole, boiled	3½-oz. serving	69
(Southland) whole	4-oz. serving	80
(Stouffer's):		
Au gratin	⅓ of pkg.	135
Scalloped	⅓ of pkg.	126
POTATO & BACON, canned		
(Hormel) *Short Orders*, au gratin	7½-oz can	230
POTATO & BEEF, canned, *Dinty*		
Moore, Short Orders, hashed	1½-oz. can	250
POTATO CHIP:		
(Bachman) regular	1 oz.	160
(Featherweight) unsalted	1 oz.	160
(Frito-Lay's) natural	1 oz.	157
Lay's, sour cream & onion flavor	1 oz.	160
(Planter's) stackable	1 oz.	150
Pringle's:		
Regular	1 oz.	172
Light	1 oz.	146
POTATO & HAM, canned (Hormel)		
Short Orders, scalloped	7½-oz. can	250
*POTATO MIX:		
Au gratin:		
(Betty Crocker)	½ cup	150
(French's) *Big Tate*, tangy	½ cup	150
(Libby's) *Potato Classics*	¾ cup	130
Creamed (Betty Crocker)	½ cup	160
Hash browns (Betty Crocker) with		
onion	½ cup	150
Hickory smoke cheese		
(Betty Crocker)	½ cup	150
Julienne (Betty Crocker) with mild		
cheese sauce	½ cup	130
Mashed:		
(American Beauty)	½ cup	120
(Betty Crocker) *Buds*	½ cup	130
(French's) *Big Tate*	½ cup	140
(Pillsbury) *Hungry Jack*, flakes	½ cup	140
Scalloped:		
(Betty Crocker)	½ cup	140
(French's) *Big Tate*	½ cup	160
(Libby's) *Potato Classics*	¾ cup	130
Sour cream & chive (Betty Crocker)	½ cup	150

Food and Description	Measure or Quantity	Calories
*POTATO PANCAKE MIX		
(French's) *Big Tate*	3" pancake	43
POTATO SALAD:		
Home recipe	½ cup	181
Canned (Nalley's):		
Regular	4-oz. serving	139
German style	4-oz. serving	143
POTATO STICK (Durkee) *O & C*	1½-oz. can	231
POTATO, STUFFED, BAKED,		
frozen (Green Giant):		
With cheese flavored topping	½ potato	180
With sour cream & chives	½ potato	240
POTATO TOPPERS (Libby's)	1 T.	30
POUND CAKE (See CAKE, Pound)		
PRESERVE OR JAM (See also		
individual flavors) (Crosse &		
Blackwell)	1 T.	60
PRETZEL:		
(Bachman) regular or butter	1 oz.	110
(Featherweight) unsalted	1 piece	7
(Nabisco) *Mister Salty*, Dutch	1 piece	55
(Rokeach) *Baldies*	1 oz.	110
PRODUCT 19, cereal (Kellogg's)	¾ cup	110
PRUNE:		
Canned:		
(Del Monte):		
Moist-Pak	2 oz.	142
Stewed, solids & liq.	4 oz.	131
(Featherweight) stewed,		
water pack	½ cup	130
(Sunsweet) stewed	½ cup	120
Dried:		
(Del Monte):		
Breakfast or medium	2 oz.	151
Pitted	2 oz.	150
(Sunsweet) whole	2 oz.	130
PRUNE JUICE:		
(Del Monte)	6 fl. oz.	137
(Mott's)	6 fl. oz.	140
(Mott's) with prune pulp	6 fl. oz.	120
(Sunsweet) regular or with pulp	6 fl. oz.	130
PRUNE NECTAR, canned (Mott's)	6 fl. oz.	100
PRUNE WHIP, home recipe	½ cup	106
PUDDING OR PIE FILLING:		
Canned, regular pack:		
Banana:		
(Del Monte) *Pudding Cup*	5-oz. container	181
(Hunt's) *Snack Pack*	5-oz. container	180

Food and Description	Measure or Quantity	Calories
Butterscotch:		
(Del Monte) *Pudding Cup*	5-oz. container	184
(Hunt's) *Snack Pack*	5-oz. container	170
Chocolate:		
(Del Monte) *Pudding Cup*	5-oz. container	201
(Hunt's) *Snack Pack*	5-oz. container	180
Rice:		
(Comstock)	½ of 7½-oz. can	120
(Menner's)	½ of 7½-oz. can	120
Tapioca:		
(Del Monte) *Pudding Cup*	5-oz. container	172
(Hunt's) *Snack Pack*	5-oz. container	140
Vanilla (Del Monte)	5-oz. container	188
Canned, dietetic pack (Sego) all flavors	4-oz. serving	125
Chilled, *Swiss Miss:*		
Butterscotch, chocolate malt or vanilla	4-oz. container	150
Chocolate or double rich	4-oz. container	160
Tapioca	4-oz. container	130
Frozen (Rich's):		
Banana	3-oz. container	142
Butterscotch or vanilla	4½-oz. container	199
Chocolate	4½-oz. container	214
Mix, sweetened, regular & instant:		
Banana:		
*(Jell-O) cream:		
Regular	½ cup	161
Instant	½ cup	174
*(Royal):		
Regular	½ cup	160
Instant	½ cup	180
*Butter Pecan (Jell-O) instant	½ cup	175
Butterscotch:		
*(Jell-O):		
Regular	½ cup	172
Instant	½ cup	175
*(My-T-Fine) regular	½ cup	143
*(Royal) regular	½ cup	160
Chocolate:		
*(Jell-O) regular	½ cup	174
*(My-T-Fine) regular	½ cup	169
*(Royal) regular	½ cup	180
Coconut:		
*(Jell-O) cream, regular	½ cup	176
*(Royal) instant	½ cup	170
Custard *(Royal) regular	½ cup	150
*Flan (Royal) regular	½ cup	150

Food and Description	Measure or Quantity	Calories
Lemon:		
*(Jell-O):		
Regular	½ cup	181
Instant	½ cup	179
*(My-T-Fine) regular	½ cup	164
*(Royal) instant	½ cup	180
*Lime (Royal) Key Lime, regular	½ cup	160
*Pineapple (Jell-O) cream, regular	½ cup	176
Pistachio *(Royal) nut, instant	½ cup	170
*Raspberry (Salada) *Danish Dessert*	½ cup	130
*Rice, *Jell-O Americana*	½ cup	176
*Strawberry (Salada) *Danish Dessert*	½ cup	130
Tapioca:		
Jell-O Americana, chocolate	½ cup	173
*(My-T-Fine) vanilla	½ cup	130
*(Royal) vanilla	½ cup	160
Vanilla:		
*(Jell-O) regular	½ cup	143
*(Jell-O) French, regular	½ cup	172
*(My-T-Fine) regular	½ cup	133
*(Royal) instant	½ cup	180
*Mix, dietetic:		
Butterscotch:		
(D-Zerta)	½ cup	69
(Featherweight) artificially sweetened	½ cup	60
Chocolate:		
(D-Zerta)	½ cup	68
(Estee)	½ cup	48
(Featherweight) artificially sweetened	½ cup	60
Lemon:		
(Dia-Mel)	½ cup	53
(Estee)	½ cup	106
Vanilla:		
(D-Zerta)	½ cup	71
(Estee)	½ cup	39
(Featherweight) artificially sweetened	½ cup	60
PUFFED RICE:		
(Malt-O-Meal)	1 cup	50
(Quaker)	1 cup	55
PUFFED WHEAT:		
(Malt-O-Meal)	1 cup	50

Food and Description	Measure or Quantity	Calories
(Quaker)	1 cup	54
PUMPKIN, canned (Libby's) solid pack	½ cup	80
PUMPKIN SEED, in hull	1 oz.	116

Q

QUAIL, raw, meat & skin	4 oz.	195
QUIK (Nestlé) chocolate or strawberry	1 tsp.	45
QUISP, cereal	1⅙ cup	121

R

RADISH	2 small radishes	4
RAISIN, dried:		
(Del Monte) golden	3 oz.	287
(Sun-Maid)	3 oz.	290
RAISINS, RICE & RYE, cereal (Kellogg's)	¾ cup	140
RALSTON, cereal	¼ cup	90
RASPBERRY:		
Fresh:		
Black, trimmed	½ cup	49
Red, trimmed	½ cup	41
Frozen (Birds Eye) quick thaw	5-oz. serving	155
RASPBERRY PRESERVE OR JAM:		
Sweetened (Smucker's)	1 T.	53
Dietetic:		
(Featherweight) red	1 T.	16
(S&W) *Nutradiet,* red	1 T.	12
RASPBERRY SPREAD, low sugar (Smucker's)	1 T.	24
RAVIOLI:		
Canned, regular pack:		
(Franco-American):		
Beef, *RavioliOs*	7½-oz. serving	210
Cheese, in tomato sauce, *RavioliOs*	7½-oz. can	260
(Nalley's) beef	8-oz. serving	214
Canned, dietetic (Featherweight)		

Food and Description	Measure or Quantity	Calories
beef	8-oz. can	260
RELISH:		
Hamburger (Nalley's)	1 T.	17
Hot dog (Nalley's)	1 T.	24
Sweet (Smucker's)	1 T.	23
RENNET MIX (Junket):		
*Powder, any flavor:		
Made with skim milk	½ cup	90
Made with whole milk	½ cup	120
Tablet	1 tablet	1
RHINE WINE:		
(Great Western)	3 fl. oz.	73
(Inglenook) Navalle	3 fl. oz.	76
(Taylor)	3 fl. oz.	75
RHUBARB, cooked, sweetened	½ cup	169
RICE:		
*Brown (Uncle Ben's) parboiled, with added butter	⅔ cup	152
*White:		
(Minute Rice) instant, no added butter	⅔ cup	120
(Success) long grain	½ cooking bag	110
*White & wild (Carolina)	½ cup	90
RICE, FRIED (See also RICE MIX):		
*Canned (La Choy)	½ of 11-oz. can	192
Frozen:		
(Birds Eye)	3.7 oz.	107
(La Choy) & pork	6-oz. serving	245
***RICE, FRIED, SEASONING MIX** (Durkee)	1 cup	213
RICE KRINKLES, cereal (Post)	⅞ cup	109
RICE KRISPIES, cereal (Kellogg's)	1 cup	110
RICE MIX:		
Beef:		
*(Carolina) *Bake-It-Easy*	¼ of pkg.	110
(Minute Rice)	½ cup	149
Rice-A-Roni	⅙ of 8-oz. pkg.	129
Chicken:		
*(Carolina) *Bake-It-Easy*	¼ of pkg.	110
Rice-A-Roni	⅕ of 8-oz. pkg.	160
*Fried (Minute Rice)	½ cup	156
Long grain & wild (Uncle Ben's) with added butter	½ cup	112
*Oriental (Carolina) *Bake-It-Easy*	½ of pkg.	120
Spanish:		
*(Carolina) *Bake-It-Easy*	¼ of pkg.	110
*(Minute Rice)	½ cup	150
Rice-A-Roni	⅙ of 7½-oz. pkg.	124

Food and Description	Measure or Quantity	Calories
RICE, SPANISH, canned:		
Canned, regular:		
(Comstock)	½ of 7½-oz. can	140
(Menner's)	½ of 7½-oz. can	140
Canned, dietetic (Featherweight) low sodium	7½ oz.	140
Frozen (Birds Eye)	3.7 oz.	122
RICE & VEGETABLE, frozen:		
(Birds Eye):		
French style	3.7 oz.	117
Peas with mushrooms	2⅓ oz.	109
(Green Giant) *Rice Originals*		
& broccoli in cheese sauce	½ cup	140
Country style French	½ cup	160
Festive	½ cup	140
Medley	½ cup	120
Verdi	½ cup	130
RICE WINE:		
Chinese, 20.7% alcohol	1 fl. oz.	38
Japanese, 10.6% alcohol	1 fl. oz.	72
RIESLING WINE, Grey (Inglenook)	3 fl. oz.	60
ROCK & RYE (Mr. Boston)	1 fl. oz.	74
ROE, baked or broiled, cod & shad	4 oz.	143
ROLL OR BUN:		
Commercial type, non-frozen:		
Biscuit (Wonder)	1¼-oz. piece	99
Brown & serve (Wonder)		
Gem Style	1-oz. piece	72
Club (Pepperidge Farm)	1⅓-oz. piece	100
Crescent (Pepperidge Farm) butter	1-oz. piece	110
Croissant (Pepperidge Farm):		
Butter, cinnamon or honey-sesame	2-oz. piece	200
Chocolate	2.4-oz. piece	260
Walnut	2-oz. piece	210
Dinner:		
Home Pride	1-oz. piece	85
(Pepperidge Farm)	.7-oz. piece	60
(Wonder)	1¼-oz. piece	99
Finger (Pepperidge Farm) sesame or poppy	.6-oz. piece	60
Frankfurter:		
(Arnold) Hot Dog	1.3-oz. piece	110
(Pepperidge Farm)	1¾-oz. piece	110
(Wonder)	2-oz. piece	157
French:		
(Arnold) *Francisco*, Sourdough	1.1-oz. piece	90

Food and Description	Measure or Quantity	Calories
(Pepperidge Farm):		
Small	1⅓-oz. piece	110
Large	3-oz. piece	240
Golden Twist (Pepperidge Farm)	1-oz. piece	120
Hamburger:		
(Arnold)	1.4-oz. piece	110
(Pepperidge Farm)	1½-oz. piece	130
Roman Meal	1.8-oz. piece	193
Hoggie (Wonder)	6-oz. piece	465
Honey (Hostess) glazed	3¾-oz. piece	422
Kaiser (Wonder)	6-oz. piece	465
Old fashioned (Pepperidge Farm)	.6-oz. piece	60
Pan (Wonder)	1¼-oz. piece	99
Parkerhouse (Pepperidge Farm)	.6-oz. piece	60
Party (Pepperidge Farm)	.4-oz. piece	45
Sandwich (Arnold) soft	1.3-oz. piece	110
Soft (Pepperidge Farm)	1¼-oz. piece	110
Frozen:		
Apple crunch (Sara Lee)	1-oz. piece	102
Caramel pecan (Sara Lee)	1.3-oz. piece	161
Cinnamon (Sara Lee)	.9-oz. piece	100
Croissant (Sara Lee)	.9-oz. piece	109
Crumb (Sara Lee):		
Blueberry	1¾-oz. piece	169
French	1¾-oz. piece	188
Danish (Sara Lee):		
Apple	1.3-oz. piece	120
Cheese	1.3-oz. piece	130
Cheese Country	1½-oz. piece	146
Cinnamon Raisin	1.3-oz. piece	147
Pecan	1.3-oz. piece	148
Honey:		
(Morton):		
Regular	2½-oz. piece	231
Mini	1.3-oz. piece	133
(Sara Lee)	1-oz. piece	109
ROLL OR BUN DOUGH:		
*Frozen (Rich's):		
Cinnamon	2¼-oz. piece	173
Frankfurter	1 piece	136
Hamburger, regular	1 piece	134
Onion, regular	1 piece	155
Parkerhouse	1 piece	82
Refrigerated (Pillsbury):		
Caramel danish, with nuts	1 piece	150
Cinnamon with icing, *Ballard*	1 piece	100
Cinnamon raisin danish	1 piece	135
Crescent	1 piece	200

Food and Description	Measure or Quantity	Calories
White, Bakery Style	1 piece	90
*ROLL MIX, HOT (Pillsbury)	1 piece	95
ROMAN MEAL cereal	⅓ cup	103
ROSEMARY LEAVES (French's)	1 tsp.	5
ROSÉ WINE:		
(Great Western)	3 fl. oz.	80
(Inglenook) Gamay or Vintage	3 fl. oz.	60
(Paul Masson):		
Regular, 11.8% alcohol	3 fl. oz.	76
Light, 7.1% alcohol	3 fl. oz.	49
RUM EXTRACT (Durkee) imitation	1 tsp.	14
RUTABAGA:		
Canned (Sunshine) solids & liq.	½ cup	32
Frozen (Southland)	4 oz.	50

S

Food and Description	Measure or Quantity	Calories
SAFFLOWER SEED, in hull	1 oz.	89
SAGE (French's)	1 tsp.	4
SAKE WINE	1 fl. oz.	39
SALAD CRUNCHIES (Libby's)	1 T.	35
SALAD DRESSING:		
Regular:		
Bacon (Seven Seas) creamy	1 T.	60
Bleu or blue cheese:		
(Bernstein) Danish	1 T.	60
(Wish-Bone) chunky	1 T.	70
Caesar:		
(Pfeiffer)	1 T.	70
(Seven Seas) *Viva*	1 T.	60
(Wish-Bone)	1 T.	80
Capri (Seven Seas)	1 T.	70
Cucumber (Wish-Bone)	1 T.	80
French:		
(Bernstein's) creamy	1 T.	56
(Seven Seas) creamy	1 T.	60
(Wish-Bone) any type	1 T.	60
Garlic (Wish-Bone) creamy	1 T.	80
Green Goddess:		
(Seven Seas)	1 T.	60
(Wish-Bone)	1 T.	70
Herb & spice (Seven Seas)	1 T.	60
Italian:		
(Bernstein's)	1 T.	50
(Pfeiffer) chef	1 T.	60

Food and Description	Measure or Quantity	Calories
(Seven Seas)	1 T.	70
(Wish-Bone) any type	1 T.	80
Red wine vinegar & oil		
(Seven Seas)	1 T.	60
Roquefort:		
(Bernstein's)	1 T.	65
(Marie's)	1 T.	105
Russian:		
(Pfeiffer)	1 T.	65
(Wish-Bone)	1 T.	50
Spin Blend (Hellmann's)	1 T.	57
Thousand Island:		
(Pfeiffer)	1 T.	65
(Wish-Bone)	1 T.	70
Vinaigrette (Bernstein's) French	1 T.	49
Dietetic:		
Bleu or blue cheese:		
(Featherweight) imitation	1 T.	4
(Tillie Lewis) *Tasti-Diet*	1 T.	12
(Walden Farms) chunky	1 T.	27
(Wish-Bone)	1 T.	40
Caesar:		
(Estee) garlic	1 T.	4
(Featherweight) creamy	1 T.	14
Cucumber (Featherweight) creamy	1 T.	12
Cucumber & onion		
(Featherweight) creamy	1 T.	4
French:		
(Featherweight) low calorie	1 T.	6
(Tillie Lewis) *Tasti-Diet*	1 T.	6
(Walden Farms) chunky	1 T.	33
(Wish-Bone)	1 T.	30
Herb & Spice (Featherweight)	1 T.	6
Italian:		
(Estee) spicy	1 T.	4
(Featherweight)	1 T.	4
(Tillie Lewis) *Tasti-Diet*	1 T.	2
(Weight Watchers)	1 T.	50
(Wish-Bone)	1 T.	30
Onion N' Chive (Wish-Bone)	1 T.	40
Red wine/vinegar (Featherweight)	1 T.	6
Russian:		
(Featherweight) creamy	1 T.	6
(Tillie Lewis) *Tasti-Diet*	1 T.	6
(Weight Watchers)	1 T.	50
(Wish-Bone)	1 T.	25
Thousand Island:		
(Walden Farms)	1 T.	24

Food and Description	Measure or Quantity	Calories
(Weight Watchers)	1 T.	50
(Wish-Bone)	1 T.	25
2-Calorie Low Sodium		
(Featherweight)	1 T.	2
Whipped (Tillie Lewis) *Tasti-Diet*	1 T.	18
SALAD DRESSING MIX:		
*Regular (Good Seasons):		
Bleu or blue cheese	1 T.	91
Buttermilk Farm Style	1 T.	63
Farm style	1 T.	54
French:		
Regular	1 T.	97
Old fashioned	1 T.	84
Garlic, regular or cheese	1 T.	91
Italian, regular or cheese	1 T.	90
Onion	1 T.	85
Dietetic:		
*Blue cheese (Weight Watchers)	1 T.	10
*French (Weight Watchers)	1 T.	4
Garlic (Dia-Mel)	½-oz. pkg.	21
Italian:		
*(Good Seasons)	1 T.	8
*(Weight Watchers):		
Regular	1 T.	2
Creamy	1 T.	4
*Russian (Weight Watchers)	1 T.	4
*Thousand Island (Weight Watchers)	1 T.	12
SALAMI:		
(Hormel):		
Genoa, sliced	1-oz. slice	126
Hard, sliced	1-oz. slice	117
(Oscar Mayer):		
For beer	.8-oz. slice	54
For beer, beef	.8-oz. slice	76
Cotto	.8-oz. slice	52
Hard	.3-oz. slice	33
(Swift) Genoa	1-oz. serving	114
(Vienna) beef	1-oz. serving	79
SALISBURY STEAK:		
Canned (Morton House)	6¼-oz. serving	160
Frozen:		
(Banquet):		
Buffet Supper	2-lb. pkg.	1454
Man Pleaser	19-oz. dinner	873
(Green Giant) with gravy, oven bake	7-oz serving	210

Food and Description	Measure or Quantity	Calories
(Swanson):		
Regular, with gravy	10-oz. entree	410
Hungry Man	17-oz. dinner	780
3-course	16-oz. dinner	500
TV Brand	11½-oz. dinner	430
(Stouffer's) with onion gravy	12-oz. pkg.	500
SALMON:		
Baked or broiled	6¾" × 2½" × 1"	264
Canned, regular pack:		
Keta (Bumble Bee) solids & liq.	½ cup	153
Pink or Humpback:		
(Bumble Bee) solids & liq.	½ cup	155
(Del Monte)	7¾-oz. can	290
(Libby's)	7¾-oz. can	310
Sockeye or Red or Blueback:		
(Bumble Bee) solids & liq.	½ cup	188
(Del Monte)	7¾-oz. can	330
(Libby's)	7¾-oz. can	380
Canned, dietetic (S&W) *Nutradiet*, low sodium	½ cup	188
SALMON, SMOKED (Vita):		
Lox, drained	4-oz. jar	136
Nova, drained	4-oz. can	221
SALT:		
(Morton) *Lite Salt*	1 tsp.	0
(Morton) Table	1 tsp.	0
Substitute:		
(Adolph's):		
Plain	1 tsp.	1
Seasoned	1 tsp.	6
(Morton) plain	1 tsp.	Tr.
Salt It (Dia-Mel)	1 tsp.	0
SANDWICH SPREAD:		
(Hellmann's)	1 T.	65
(Oscar Mayer)	1-oz. serving	68
SANGRIA (Taylor)	3 fl. oz.	99
SARDINE, canned:		
Atlantic (Del Monte) with tomato sauce	7½-oz. can	319
Imported (Underwood) in mustard or tomato sauce	3¾-oz. can	230
Norwegian, *King Oscar Brand*:		
In mustard or tomato sauce	3¾-oz. can	240
In oil, drained	3-oz. can	260
SAUCE:		
Regular pack:		
A-1	1 T.	12

Food and Description	Measure or Quantity	Calories
Barbecue:		
Chris & Pitt's	1 T.	15
(French's) regular or smoky	1 T.	25
(Gold's)	1 T.	16
Open Pit (General Foods) original, hot n' spicy or smoke flavor	1T.	24
Chili (See CHILI SAUCE)		
Cocktail:		
(Gold's)	1 T.	31
(Pfeiffer)	1-oz. serving	100
Escoffier Sauce Diable	1 T.	20
Escoffier Sauce Robert	1 T.	20
Famous Sauce	1 T.	69
Hot, *Frank's*	1 tsp.	1
Italian:		
(Contadina)	4 oz.	71
(Ragu) red cooking	3½-oz. serving	45
Salsa Mexicana (Contadina)	4 fl. oz.	38
Salsa Picante (Del Monte)	¼ cup	12
Salsa Roja (Del Monte)	¼ cup	18
Seafood cocktail (Del Monte)	1 T.	21
Soy:		
(Gold's)	1 T.	10
(Kikkoman)	1 T.	9
(La Choy)	1 T.	8
Spare rib (Gold's)	1 T.	51
Steak (Dawn Fresh) with mushrooms	1-oz. serving	9
Steak Supreme	1 T.	20
Sweet & sour:		
(Contadina)	4 fl. oz.	154
(La Choy)	1-oz. serving	51
Swiss steak (Carnation)	2-oz. serving	20
Taco:		
(Del Monte):		
Hot	¼ cup	16
Mild	¼ cup	14
Old El Paso	1-oz. serving	11
(Ortega)	1 T.	22
Tartar:		
(Hellmann's)	1 T.	73
(Nalley's);	1 T.	89
Teriyaki (Kikkoman)	1 T.	16
V-8	1-oz. serving	25
White, medium	¼ cup	103
Worcestershire:		
(French's) regular or smoky	1 T.	10

Food and Description	Measure or Quantity	Calories
(Gold's)	1 T.	42
SAUCE MIX:		
Regular:		
A la King (Durkee)	1-oz. pkg.	133
*Cheese:		
(Durkee)	½ cup	168
(French's)	½ cup	160
Hollandaise:		
(Durkee)	1-oz. pkg.	173
*(French's)	1 T.	15
Sour cream:		
*(Durkee)	⅔ cup	214
*(French's)	2½ T.	60
*Sweet & sour (Durkee)	1 cup	230
*Teriyaki (French's)	1 T.	17
*White (Durkee)	1 cup	238
*Dietetic (Weight Watchers) lemon butter	1 T.	8
SAUERKRAUT:		
(Claussen) drained	½ cup	16
(Del Monte) solids & liq.	1 cup	55
(Silver Floss):		
Regular, solids & liq.	½ cup	30
Krispy Kraut, solids & liq.	½ cup	25
SAUSAGE:		
*Brown 'n Serve (Swift) original	.8-oz. link	77
Italian style (Best's Kosher; Oscherwitz)	3-oz. link	271
Polish-style:		
(Best's Kosher; Oscherwitz)	3-oz. link	271
(Vienna) beer	3-oz. link	240
Pork:		
*(Hormel) *Little Sizzlers*	1 link	65
(Jimmy Dean)	2-oz. serving	227
*(Oscar Mayer) *Little Friers*	.6-oz. link	64
Smoked:		
(Eckrich) beef, *Smok-Y-Links*	.8-oz. link	75
(Hormel) pork	3-oz. serving	295
(Oscar Mayer) beef	1½-oz. link	132
(Vienna)	2½-oz. serving	196
*Turkey (Louis Rich) links or tube	1-oz. serving	45
SAUSAGE SANDWICH, frozen (Stouffer's)	8¼ oz.	470
SAUTERNE:		
(Great Western)	3 fl. oz.	79
(Taylor)	3 fl. oz.	81
SCALLOP:		
Steamed	4-oz. serving	127

Food and Description	Measure or Quantity	Calories
Frozen (Mrs. Paul's):		
Breaded & fried	3½-oz. serving	201
With butter & cheese	7-oz. pkg.	267
SCHAV SOUP (Gold's)	8-oz. serving	11
SCHNAPPS, APPLE (Mr. Boston)	1 fl. oz.	75
SCHNAPPS, PEPPERMINT		
(Mr. Boston)	1 fl. oz.	115
SCREWDRIVER COCKTAIL:		
Canned (Mr. Boston) 12½% alcohol	3 fl. oz.	111
Mix, dry (Bar-Tender's)	1 serving	70
SEAFOOD PLATTER, frozen (Mrs. Paul's) breaded, fried	4½-oz. serving	254
SEGO **DIET FOOD,** canned, any flavor	10-fl.-oz. can	225
SELTZER (Canada Dry)	Any quantity	0
SERUTAN:		
Toasted granules	1 tsp.	6
Concentrated powder	1 tsp.	5
Fruit-flavored powder	1 tsp.	6
SESAME SEEDS (French's)	1 tsp.	9
SHAD, CREOLE	4-oz. serving	172
SHAKE 'N BAKE:		
Chicken, original	1 pkg.	501
Crispy country mild	1 pkg.	309
Fish	2-oz. pkg.	232
Italian	1 pkg.	289
Pork:		
Original	1 pkg.	253
Barbecue	1 pkg.	306
SHERBET:		
(Baskin-Robbins):		
Daiquiri Ice	1 scoop	99
Orange	1 scoop	84
(Meadow Gold) orange	¼ pint	120
SHERRY:		
Cocktail (Gold Seal)	3 fl. oz.	122
Cream:		
(Great Western) Solera	3 fl. oz.	141
(Taylor)	3 fl. oz.	138
Dry:		
(Italian Swiss Colony) *Gold Medal*	3 fl. oz.	104
(Williams & Humbert)	3 fl. oz.	120
Dry Sack (Williams & Humbert)	3 fl. oz.	120
SHREDDED WHEAT:		
(Nabisco):		
Regular size	¾-oz. biscuit	90
Spoon Size	⅔ cup	110

Food and Description	Measure or Quantity	Calories
(Quaker)	1 biscuit	52
SHRIMP:		
Canned:		
(Bumble Bee) solids & liq.	4½-oz. can	90
(Icy Point) cocktail	4½-oz. can	148
Frozen (Mrs. Paul's) fried	3-oz. serving	198
SHRIMP DINNER, frozen:		
(Stouffer's) Newburg	6½ oz.	300
(Van de Kamp's)	10-oz. dinner	370
SHRIMP PUFF (Durkee)	1 piece	44
SHRIMP STICKS, frozen (Mrs. Paul's)	.8-oz. stick	48
SLENDER (Carnation):		
Bar	1 bar	135
Dry	1 packet	110
Liquid	10-fl.-oz. can	220
SLOPPY HOT DOG SEASONING MIX (French's)	1½-oz. pkg.	160
SLOPPY JOE:		
Canned:		
(Hormel) *Short Orders*	7½-oz. can	340
(Libby's):		
Beef	⅓ cup	110
Pork	⅓ cup	120
(Morton House) beef	5-oz. serving	240
Frozen (Banquet) *Cookin' Bag*	5-oz. bag	199
SLOPPY JOE SEASONING MIX:		
*(Durkee):		
Regular flavor	1¼ cups	726
Pizza flavor	1¼ cups	746
(French's)	1½-oz. pkg.	128
SNACK BAR (Pepperidge Farm):		
Apple nut, apricot-raspberry or blueberry	1.7-oz. piece	170
Brownie nut or date nut	1½-oz. piece	190
Chocolate chip or coconut macaroon	1½-oz. piece	210
Raisin spice	1½-oz. piece	180
SNO BALL (Hostess)	1 cake	149
SOAVE WINE (Antinori)	3 fl. oz.	84
SOFT DRINK:		
Sweetened:		
Birch beer (Canada Dry)	6 fl. oz.	82
Bitter lemon:		
(Canada Dry)	6 fl. oz.	75
(Schweppes)	6 fl. oz.	84
Bubble Up	6 fl. oz.	73
Cactus Cooler (Canada Dry)	6 fl. oz.	90
Cherry:		
(Canada Dry) wild	6 fl. oz.	98

Food and Description	Measure or Quantity	Calories
(Shasta) black	6 fl. oz.	79
Chocolate (Yoo-Hoo)	6 fl. oz.	108
Club (any brand)	6 fl. oz.	0
Cola:		
Coca-Cola:		
Regular	6 fl. oz.	72
Caffeine-free	6 fl. oz.	76
Jamaica (Canada Dry)	6 fl. oz.	82
Pepsi-Cola, regular or *Pepsi Free*	6 fl. oz.	79
(Royal Crown)	6 fl. oz.	78
(Shasta)	6 fl. oz.	72
Collins mix (Canada Dry)	6 fl. oz.	60
Cream:		
(Canada Dry) vanilla	6 fl. oz.	97
(Schweppes) red	6 fl. oz.	86
(Shasta)	6 fl. oz.	75
Dr. Pepper	6 fl. oz.	75
Fruit Punch:		
(Nehi)	6 fl. oz.	91
(Shasta)	6 fl. oz.	84
Ginger ale:		
(Canada Dry) regular	6 fl. oz.	68
(Fanta)	6 fl. oz.	63
(Shasta)	6 fl. oz.	59
Ginger beer (Schweppes)	6 fl. oz.	72
Grape:		
(Canada Dry) concord	6 fl. oz.	97
(Fanta)	6 fl. oz.	86
(Hi-C)	6 fl. oz.	78
(Nehi)	6 fl. oz.	87
(Schweppes)	6 fl. oz.	97
(Welch's) sparkling	6 fl. oz.	90
Half & half (Canada Dry)	6 fl. oz.	82
Hi-Spot (Canada Dry)	6 fl. oz.	75
Island Lime (Canada Dry)	6 fl. oz.	97
Lemon (Hi-C)	6 fl. oz.	75
Lemon-lime (Shasta)	6 fl. oz.	69
Mello Yello	6 fl. oz.	86
Mountain Dew	6 fl. oz.	89
Mr. PiBB	6 fl. oz.	71
Orange:		
(Canada Dry) *Sunripe*	6 fl. oz.	97
(Fanta)	6 fl. oz.	88
(Hi-C)	6 fl. oz.	77
(Sunkist)	6 fl. oz.	96
(Welch's)	6 fl. oz.	90
Peach (Nehi)	6 fl. oz.	92
Pineapple (Canada Dry)	6 fl. oz.	82

Food and Description	Measure or Quantity	Calories
Purple Passion (Canada Dry)	6 fl. oz.	90
Quinine or Tonic Water:		
(Canada Dry)	6 fl. oz.	67
(Schweppes)	6 fl. oz.	66
Rondo (Schweppes)	6 fl. oz.	77
Root Beer:		
Barrelhead (Canada Dry)	6 fl. oz.	82
(Dad's)	6 fl. oz.	83
(Nehi)	6 fl. oz.	87
On Tap	6 fl. oz.	81
Rooti (Canada Dry)	6 fl. oz.	79
(Shasta) draft	6 fl. oz.	75
Seven-Up	6 fl. oz.	72
Sprite	6 fl. oz.	71
Strawberry:		
(Canada Dry) California	6 fl. oz.	90
(Shasta)	6 fl. oz.	72
(Welch's)	6 fl. oz.	90
Tahitian Treat (Canada Dry)	6 fl. oz.	97
Teem	6 fl. oz.	74
Upper 10 (Royal Crown)	6 fl. oz.	76
Whiskey Sour (Canada Dry)	6 fl. oz.	67
Wink (Canada Dry)	6 fl. oz.	90
Dietetic or low calorie:		
Bubble Up	6 fl. oz.	1
Cherry:		
(No-Cal) black	6 fl. oz.	1
(Shasta) black	6 fl. oz.	<1
Chocolate (No-Cal)	6 fl. oz.	1
Coffee (No-Cal)	6 fl. oz.	1
Cola:		
(Canada Dry)	6 fl. oz.	0
Coca-Cola, regular or caffeine free	6 fl. oz.	<1
Diet-Rite	6 fl. oz.	<1
(No-Cal)	6 fl. oz.	0
Pepsi, diet, light or free	6 fl. oz.	<1
(Shasta) regular or cherry	6 fl. oz.	<1
Cream:		
(No-Cal)	6 fl. oz.	0
(Shasta)	6 fl. oz.	<1
Dr. Pepper	6 fl. oz.	<2
Fresca	6 fl. oz.	2
Ginger Ale:		
(Canada Dry)	6 fl. oz.	1
(No-Cal)	6 fl. oz.	0
(Shasta)	6 fl. oz.	<1
Grape (Shasta)	6 fl. oz.	<1

Food and Description	Measure or Quantity	Calories
Grapefruit (Shasta)	6 fl. oz.	<1
Lemon-lime (No-Cal)	6 fl. oz.	1
Mr. PiBB	6 fl. oz.	<1
Orange:		
(Canada Dry)	6 fl. oz.	1
(No-Cal)	6 fl. oz.	1
(Shasta)	6 fl. oz.	<1
Quinine or Tonic (No-Cal)	6 fl. oz.	3
RC 100 (Royal Crown) caffeine free	6 fl. oz.	<1
Root Beer:		
Barrelhead (Canada Dry)	6 fl. oz.	1
(Dad's)	6 fl. oz.	<1
(No-Cal)	6 fl. oz.	1
(Ramblin')	6 fl. oz.	<1
(Shasta) draft	6 fl. oz.	<1
Seven-Up	6 fl. oz.	2
Sprite	6 fl. oz.	1
Strawberry (Shasta)	6 fl. oz.	<1
Tab, regular or caffeine free	6 fl. oz.	<1
SOLE, frozen:		
(Mrs. Paul's):		
Fillets, breaded & fried	4-oz. serving	225
Fillets, with lemon butter	4½-oz. serving	155
(Van de Kamp's) batter dipped, french fried	1 piece	140
(Weight Watchers) in lemon sauce	9¼-oz. meal	201
SOUP:		
Canned, regular pack:		
*Asparagus (Campbell) condensed, cream of	8 oz.	90
Bean:		
(Campbell):		
Chunky, with ham, old fashioned	11-oz. can	290
*Condensed, with bacon	8 oz.	150
*Semi-condensed, *Soup For One*, with ham	11 oz.	220
(Grandma Brown's)	8 oz.	182
Bean, black:		
*(Campbell) condensed	8 oz.	110
(Crosse & Blackwell)	6½ oz.	80
Beef:		
(Campbell):		
Chunky:		
Regular	10¾-oz. can	190
With noodles	10¾-oz. can	300

122

Food and Description	Measure or Quantity	Calories
*Condensed:		
Regular	8 oz.	80
Broth:		
Plain	8 oz.	16
& barley	8 oz.	60
& noodles	8 oz.	60
Consomme	8 oz.	25
Mushroom	8 oz.	70
Noodle	8 oz.	70
Teriyaki	8 oz.	70
(College Inn) broth	1 cup	18
(Swanson)	7½-oz. can	20
Celery:		
*(Campbell) condensed, cream of	8 oz.	100
*(Rokeach) condensed:		
Prepared with milk	10 oz.	190
Prepared with water	10 oz.	90
*Cheddar cheese (Campbell)	8 oz.	130
Chicken:		
(Campbell):		
Chunky:		
Regular	10¾-oz. can	200
Old fashioned	10¾-oz. can	170
& rice	19-oz. can	280
Vegetable	19-oz. can	340
*Condensed:		
Alphabet	8 oz.	80
Broth:		
Plain	8 oz.	35
& rice	8 oz.	50
Cream of	8 oz.	110
Gumbo	8 oz.	60
Mushroom, creamy	8 oz.	110
NoodleOs	8 oz.	70
Oriental	8 oz.	50
& rice	8 oz.	60
Vegetable	8 oz.	70
*Semi-condensed, *Soup For One:*		
& noodles, golden	11 oz.	130
Vegetable, full flavored	11 oz.	120
(College Inn) broth	1 cup	35
(Swanson) broth	7¼-oz. can	35
Chili beef (Campbell):		
Chunky	11-oz. can	300
*Condensed	8 oz.	130

Food and Description	Measure or Quantity	Calories
Chowder:		
Beef'n vegetable (Hormel)	7½-oz. can	120
Chicken'n corn (Hormel)	7½-oz. can	130
Clam:		
Manhattan style:		
(Campbell):		
Chunky	18-oz. can	300
*Condensed	8 oz.	70
(Crosse & Blackwell)	6½ oz.	50
New England style:		
*(Campbell):		
Condensed:		
Made with milk	8 oz.	150
Made with water	8 oz.	80
Semi-condensed, *Soup For One*:		
Made with milk	11 oz.	200
Made with water	11 oz.	130
(Crosse & Blackwell)	6½ oz.	90
Ham'n potato (Hormel)	7½-oz. can	130
Consomme madrilene (Crosse & Blackwell)	6½ oz.	25
Crab (Crosse & Blackwell)	6½ oz.	50
Gazpacho:		
*(Campbell's) condensed	8 oz.	50
(Crosse & Blackwell)	6½ oz.	30
Ham'n butter bean (Campbell) *Chunky*	10¾-oz. can	280
Lentil (Crosse & Blackwell) with ham	6½ oz.	80
*Meatball alphabet (Campbell) condensed	8 oz.	100
Mexicali bean (Campbell) *Chunky*	19½-oz. can	420
Minestrone:		
(Campbell):		
Chunky	18-oz. can	300
*Condensed	8 oz.	80
(Crosse & Blackwell)	6½ oz.	90
Mushroom:		
*(Campbell):		
Condensed:		
Cream of	8 oz.	100
Golden	8 oz.	80
Semi-condensed, *Soup For One*, cream of, savory	11oz.	180
(Crosse & Blackwell) cream of, bisque	6½ oz.	90

Food and Description	Measure or Quantity	Calories
*(Rokeach) cream of:		
Prepared with milk	10 oz.	240
Prepared with water	10 oz.	150
*Mushroom barley (Campbell's)	8 oz.	80
*Noodle (Campbell):		
Curley noodle with chicken	8 oz.	70
& ground beef	8 oz.	90
*Onion (Campbell):		
Regular	8 oz.	70
Cream of:		
Made with water	8 oz.	100
Made with water & milk	8 oz.	160
*Oyster stew (Campbell):		
Made with milk	8 oz.	140
Made with water	8 oz.	70
*Pea, green (Campbell)	8 oz.	150
Pea, split:		
(Campbell):		
Chunky, with ham	18-oz. can	400
*Condensed, with ham & bacon	8 oz.	170
(Grandma Brown's)	8 oz.	184
*Pepper pot (Campbell)	8 oz.	90
*Potato (Campbell) cream of:		
Made with water	8 oz.	70
Made with water & milk	8 oz.	130
*Scotch broth (Campbell)	8 oz.	80
Shrimp:		
*(Campbell) condensed, cream of:		
Made with milk	8 oz.	160
Made with water	8 oz.	90
(Crosse & Blackwell) cream of	6½ oz.	90
Sirloin burger (Campbell) *Chunky*	19-oz. can	400
Steak & potato (Campbell) *Chunky*	19-oz. can	340
Tomato:		
*(Campbell):		
Condensed:		
Regular:		
Made with milk	8 oz.	160
Made with water	8 oz.	90
Bisque	8 oz.	120
& rice, old fashioned	8 oz.	110
Semi-condensed, *Soup For One*, Royale	11 oz.	180
*(Rokeach):		
Made with milk	10 oz.	190

Food and Description	Measure or Quantity	Calories
Made with water	10 oz.	90
Turkey (Campbell):		
Chunky	18¾-oz. can	360
*Condensed:		
Noodle	8 oz.	60
Vegetable	8 oz.	70
Vegetable:		
(Campbell):		
Chunky:		
Regular	19-oz. can	260
Beef, old fashioned	19-oz. can	360
Mediterranean	19-oz. can	340
*Condensed:		
Regular	8 oz.	80
Beef	8 oz.	70
Vegetarian	8 oz.	70
*Semi-condensed, *Soup For One*:		
Barley, with beef	11 oz.	150
Old world	11 oz.	130
*(Rokeach) vegetarian	10 oz.	90
Vichyssoise (Crosse & Blackwell) cream of	6½ oz.	70
*Won ton (Campbell)	8 oz.	40
Canned, dietetic pack:		
Beef:		
(Campbell) & mushroom, low sodium	10¾-oz. can	200
(Dia-Mel) & noodle	8 oz.	70
Chicken:		
(Campbell) low sodium:		
Chunky	7½-oz. can	150
With noodles	10¾-oz. can	180
Vegetable	10¾-oz. can	240
*(Dia-Mel) broth	8 oz.	18
Corn (Campbell) low sodium	10¾-oz. can	190
Mushroom (Campbell) cream of, low sodium	7¼-oz. can	130
Pea, green (Campbell) low sodium	7½-oz. can	160
Pea, split (Campbell) low sodium	10¾-oz. can	220
Tomato (Campbell) low sodium:		
Regular	7¼-oz. can	140
With tomato pieces	10½-oz. can	200
Turkey (Campbell) & noodle, low sodium	7¼-oz. can	70
Vegetable (Campbell) low sodium:		
Regular	7¼-oz. can	90

Food and Description	Measure or Quantity	Calories
Chunky	10¾-oz. can	180
Frozen:		
*Barley & mushroom (Mother's Own)	8 oz.	50
Chowder, Clam, New England style (Stouffer's)	8 oz.	200
Pea, split:		
*(Mother's Own)	8 oz.	130
(Stouffer's)	8¼ oz.	190
Spinach (Stouffer's) cream of	8 oz.	230
*Vegetable (Mother's Own)	8 oz.	40
*Won ton (La Choy)	1 cup	92
Mix, regular:		
Beef:		
*Carmel Kosher	6 fl. oz.	12
*(Lipton):		
Cup-A-Soup, regular and noodle	6 fl. oz.	50
Lots-A-Noodles	7 fl. oz.	120
*(Weight Watchers) broth	6 fl. oz.	10
*Chicken:		
Carmel Kosher	6 fl. oz.	12
(Lipton):		
Regular	8 fl. oz.	60
Cup-A-Broth	6 fl. oz.	25
Cup-A-Soup:		
Regular:		
Cream of	6 fl. oz.	80
& rice	6 fl. oz.	45
& vegetable	6 fl. oz.	40
Country style:		
Hearty	6 fl. oz.	70
Supreme	6 fl. oz.	100
Lots-A-Noodles	7 fl. oz.	130
Noodle Soup:		
With chicken broth	8 fl. oz.	60
With chicken meat	8 fl. oz.	50
Giggle Noodle	8 fl. oz.	80
Ripple Noodle	8 fl. oz.	80
*Mushroom:		
Carmel Kosher	6 fl. oz.	12
(Lipton):		
Regular:		
Beef	8 fl. oz.	40
Onion	8 fl. oz.	40
Cup-A-Soup, cream of	6 fl. oz.	80
*Onion:		
Carmel Kosher	6 fl. oz.	12

Food and Description	Measure or Quantity	Calories
(Lipton):		
Regular:		
Plain	8 fl. oz.	35
Beefy	8 fl. oz.	30
Cup-A-Soup	6 fl. oz.	30
*Oriental (Lipton) *Cup-A-Soup*, *Lots-A-Noodles*	7 fl. oz.	130
*Pea, green (Lipton) *Cup-A-Soup*	6 fl. oz.	120
*Pea, Virginia (Lipton) *Cup-A-Soup*, Country Style	6 fl. oz.	140
*Tomato (Lipton) *Cup-A-Soup*	6 fl. oz.	80
*Vegetable (Lipton):		
Regular:		
Beef	8 fl. oz.	50
Country	8 fl. oz.	80
Cup-A-Soup:		
Regular:		
Beef	6 fl. oz.	50
Spring	6 fl. oz.	40
Country Style, harvest	6 fl. oz.	100
Lots-A-Noodles, garden	7 fl. oz.	130
(Southland) frozen	⅓ of 16-oz. pkg.	60
SOUP GREENS (Durkee)	2½-oz. jar	216
SOUTHERN COMFORT:		
86 proof	1 fl. oz.	84
100 proof	1 fl. oz.	96
SOYBEAN CURD or TOFU	2¾″ × 1½″ × 1″cake	86
SOYBEAN or NUT:		
Dry roasted (*Soy Ahoy; Soy Town*)	1 oz.	139
Oil roasted (*Soy Ahoy; Soy Town*) plain, barbecue or garlic flavored	1 oz.	152
SPAGHETTI:		
Cooked:		
8-10 minutes, "Al Dente"	1 cup	216
14-20 minutes, tender	1 cup	155
Canned:		
(Franco-American):		
With meatballs in tomato sauce	7⅜-oz. can	210
With meatballs in tomato sauce, *SpaghettiOs*	7⅜-oz. can	220
In meat sauce	7½-oz. can	220
With sliced franks in tomato sauce, *SpaghettiOs*	7⅜-oz. can	220
In tomato sauce with cheese	7⅜-oz. can	180
(Hormel) *Short Orders*, & meatballs in tomato sauce	7½-oz. can	210
(Libby's) & meatballs in tomato sauce	7½-oz. serving	189

Food and Description	Measure or Quantity	Calories
(Nalley) & meatballs	8-oz. serving	245
Dietetic (Featherweight) & meatballs	7½-oz. serving	200
Frozen:		
(Banquet):		
Buffet Supper, & meatballs	2-lb. pkg.	1127
Dinner, & meatballs	11½-oz. dinner	450
(Green Giant) & meatballs in tomato sauce	10-oz. entree	396
(Stouffer's) with meat sauce	14 oz.	445
(Swanson) *TV Brand*	12½-oz. dinner	370
SPAGHETTI SAUCE:		
Canned, regular pack:		
Marinara:		
(Prince)	4-oz. serving	80
(Ragu)	5-oz. serving	120
Meat or meat flavored:		
(Prego)	4-oz. serving	160
(Prince)	½ cup	101
(Ragu)	5-oz. serving	115
Meatless or plain:		
(Prego)	4-oz. serving	160
(Prince)	½ cup	90
(Ragu) regular	5-oz. serving	105
Mushroom:		
(Hain)	4-oz. serving	80
(Prego)	4-oz. serving	140
(Prince)	4-oz. serving	77
(Ragu)	5-oz. serving	105
Canned, dietetic pack (Featherweight)	⅔ cup	30
SPAGHETTI SAUCE MIX:		
(Durkee)	½ cup	45
(French's):		
Italian style	⅝ cup	100
With mushrooms	⅝ cup	100
(Spatini)	½ cup	84
SPAM, luncheon meat (Hormel):		
Regular or smoke flavored	1-oz. serving	88
With cheese chunks	1-oz. serving	87
Deviled	1-oz. serving	78
SPECIAL K, cereal (Kellogg's)	1 cup	110
SPINACH:		
Fresh, whole leaves	½ cup	4
Boiled	½ cup	18
Canned, regular pack (Sunshine) solids & liq.	½ cup	24

Food and Description	Measure or Quantity	Calories
Frozen:		
(Birds Eye):		
Chopped or leaf	⅓ of pkg.	28
Creamed	⅓ of pkg.	60
(Green Giant):		
Creamed	⅓ of pkg.	60
Cut leaf, in butter sauce	⅓ of pkg.	36
Harvest Fresh	4 oz.	32
(McKenzie) chopped or cut leaf	⅓ of pkg.	20
(Stouffer's) souffle	4 oz.	135
SQUASH, SUMMER:		
Yellow, boiled slices	½ cup	13
Zucchini, boiled slices	½ cup	9
Canned (Del Monte) zucchini in tomato sauce	½ cup	36
Frozen:		
(Birds Eye) zucchini	3⅓ oz.	19
(McKenzie) Crookneck	⅓ of pkg.	18
(Mrs. Paul's) zucchini, parmesan	⅓ of pkg.	84
(Southland) zucchini, sliced	⅕ of 16-oz. pkg.	15
SQUASH, WINTER:		
Acorn, baked	½ cup	56
Hubbard, baked, mashed	½ cup	51
Frozen:		
(Birds Eye)	⅓ of pkg.	43
(Southland) butternut	4 oz.	60
STEAK & GREEN PEPPERS, frozen:		
(Green Giant)	9-oz. entree	275
(Swanson)	8½-oz. entree	180
STOCK BASE (French's) beef or chicken	1 tsp.	8
STRAWBERRY:		
Fresh, capped	½ cup	26
Frozen (Birds Eye):		
Halves	⅓ of pkg.	191
Whole	¼ of pkg.	89
Whole, quick thaw	½ of pkg.	125
STRAWBERRY DRINK (Hi-C):		
Canned	6 fl. oz.	89
*Mix	6 fl. oz.	68
STRAWBERRY NECTAR (Libby's)	6 fl. oz.	60
STRAWBERRY PRESERVE OR JAM:		
Sweetened:		
(Smucker's)	1 T.	53
(Welch's)	1 T.	52
Dietetic or low calorie (See STRAWBERRY SPREAD)		

Food and Description	Measure or Quantity	Calories
STRAWBERRY SHORTCAKE cereal		
(General Mills)	1 cup	110
STRAWBERRY SPREAD, dietetic:		
(Diet Delight)	1 T.	12
(Estee)	1 T.	6
(Featherweight) artificially		
sweetened	1 T.	6
(S&W) *Nutradiet*	1 T.	12
(Welch's) Lite	1 T.	30
STUFFING MIX:		
*Chicken, *Stove Top*	½ cup	178
*Cornbread, *Stove Top*	½ cup	174
Cube (Pepperidge Farm)	1 oz.	110
Herb seasoned (Pepperidge Farm)	1 oz.	110
*Pork, *Stove Top*	½ cup	176
Seasoned (Pepperidge Farm)	1 oz.	110
White bread, *Mrs. Cubbison's*	1 oz.	101
STURGEON, smoked	4-oz. serving	169
SUCCOTASH:		
Canned:		
(Libby's) cream style	½ cup	111
(Stokely-Van Camp)	½ cup	85
Frozen (Birds Eye)	⅓ of pkg.	104
SUGAR:		
Brown	1 T.	48
Confectioners'	1 T.	30
Granulated	1 T.	46
Maple	1¾″ × 1¼″ × ½″ piece	104
SUGAR CORN POPS, cereal		
(Kellogg's)	1 cup	110
SUGAR CRISP, cereal (Post)	⅞ cup	112
SUGAR PUFFS, cereal (Malt-O-Meal)	⅞ cup	110
SUGAR SMACKS, cereal (Kellogg's)	¾ cup	110
SUGAR SUBSTITUTE:		
(Featherweight)	3 drops	0
Sprinkle Sweet (Pillsbury)	1 tsp.	2
Sweet'n-it (Dia-Mel) liquid	5 drops	0
SUNFLOWER SEED (Fisher):		
In hull, roasted, salted	1 oz.	86
Hulled, dry roasted, salted	1 oz.	164
Hulled, oil roasted, salted	1 oz.	167
SUZY Q (Hostess):		
Banana	1 cake	242
Chocolate	1 cake	237
SWEETBREADS, calf, braised	4-oz. serving	191
SWEET POTATO:		
Baked, peeled	5″ × 1″ potato	155
Canned, heavy syrup	4-oz. serving	129

Food and Description	Measure or Quantity	Calories
Frozen (Mrs. Paul's) candied, with apple	4-oz. serving	153
*SWEET & SOUR ORIENTAL, canned (La Choy):		
Chicken	7½-oz. serving	240
Pork	7½-oz. serving	260
SWISS STEAK, frozen (Swanson) *TV Brand*	10-oz. dinner	350
SWORDFISH, broiled	3″ × 3″ × ½″ steak	218
SYRUP (See also TOPPING):		
Regular:		
Apricot (Smucker's)	1 T.	50
Blackberry (Smucker's)	1 T.	50
Chocolate or chocolate-flavored:		
Bosco	1 T.	55
(Hershey's)	1 T.	52
Corn, *Karo*, dark or light	1 T.	58
Maple, *Karo*, imitation	1 T.	57
Pancake or waffle:		
(Aunt Jemima)	1 T.	53
Golden Griddle	1 T.	54
Karo	1 T.	58
Log Cabin, regular or buttered	1 T.	56
Mrs. Butterworth's	1 T.	55
Strawberry (Smucker's)	1 T.	50
Dietetic or low calorie:		
Blueberry (Featherweight)	1 T.	14
Chocolate-flavored (Diet Delight)	1 T.	8
Coffee (No-Cal)	1 T.	6
Cola (No-Cal)	1 T.	0
Maple (S&W) *Nutradiet*	1 T.	12
Pancake or waffle:		
(Aunt Jemima)	1 T.	29
(Diet Delight)	1 T.	6
(Featherweight)	1 T.	12
(Tillie Lewis) *Tasti-Diet*	1 T.	4

T

Food and Description	Measure or Quantity	Calories
TACO:		
*(Ortega)	1 taco	150
*Mix (Durkee)	½ cup	321
Shell (Ortega)	1 shell	50
TAMALE:		
Canned:		
(Hormel) beef, *Short Orders*	7½-oz. can	270

Food and Description	Measure or Quantity	Calories
(Nalley's) beef	8-oz. serving	268
Old El Paso, with chili gravy	1 tamale	116
Frozen (Hormel) beef	1 tamale	130
TAMALE PIE (Nalley's)	4-oz. serving	113
TANG:		
Grape	6 fl. oz.	93
Grapefruit	6 fl. oz.	87
Orange	6 fl. oz.	90
TANGERINE or MANDARIN ORANGE:		
Fresh (Sunkist)	1 large tangerine	39
Canned, regular pack (Del Monte) solids & liq.	5½-oz. serving	106
Canned, dietetic:		
(Diet Delight) juice pack	½ cup	50
(Featherweight) water pack	½ cup	35
(S&W) *Nutradiet*	½ cup	28
TANGERINE DRINK, canned (Hi-C)	6 fl. oz.	90
***TANGERINE JUICE,** frozen* (Minute Maid)	6 fl. oz.	85
TAPIOCA, dry, *Minute,* quick cooking	1 T.	32
TAQUITO, frozen (Van de Kamp's) beef	8 oz.	490
TARRAGON (French's)	1 tsp.	5
TASTEEOS, cereal (Ralston Purina)	1¼ cups	110
TEA:		
Bag:		
(Lipton):		
Plain	1 cup	2
Flavored	1 cup	2
Herbal:		
Almond pleasure or cinnamon apple	1 cup	2
Quietly chamomile or toasty spice	1 cup	4
(Sahadi) spearmint	1 cup	4
Instant (Lipton) lemon flavored	8 fl. oz.	4
TEAM, cereal	1 cup	110
TEA MIX, iced:		
*(Lipton) lemon & sugar flavored	1 cup	60
**Nestea,* lemon-flavored	8 fl. oz.	2
TEQUILA SUNRISE COCKTAIL, canned (Mr. Boston) 12½% alcohol	3 fl. oz.	120
***TEXTURED VEGETABLE PROTEIN,** Morningstar Farms:*		
Breakfast link	1 link	62
Breakfast patties	1 patty	109

Food and Description	Measure or Quantity	Calories
Breakfast strips	1 strip	34
Grillers	1 patty	189
THURINGER:		
(Hormel):		
Buffet	1-oz. serving	95
Old Smokehouse	1-oz. serving	100
(Louis Rich) turkey	1-oz. serving	50
(Oscar Mayer) beef	.8-oz. slice	72
TIGER TAILS (Hostess)	2¼-oz. piece	227
TOASTER CAKE OR PASTRY:		
Flavor-Kist (Schulze and Burch):		
Regular:		
All flavors except brown sugar cinnamon	1 pastry	190
Brown sugar cinnamon	1 pastry	200
Pop-Tarts (Kellogg's):		
Regular:		
Blueberry, brown sugar cinnamon & cherry	1 pastry	210
Chocolate chip & strawberry	1 pastry	200
Frosted:		
Blueberry, chocolate fudge, or strawberry	1 pastry	200
Brown sugar cinnamon, cherry, concord grape, dutch apple or raspberry	1 pastry	210
Chocolate-vanilla creme	1 pastry	220
Toastettes (Nabisco)	1 pastry	190
Toast-R-Cake (Thomas'):		
Blueberry	1 piece	116
Bran	1 piece	113
Corn	1 piece	118
TOASTIES, cereal (Post)	1¼ cup	107
TOASTY O's, cereal (Malt-O-Meal)	1¼ cups	110
TOMATO:		
Cherry, whole	4 pieces	14
Regular, whole	1 med. tomato	33
Canned, regular pack:		
(Contadina) sliced, baby	½ cup	50
(Del Monte) stewed, solids & liq.	4 oz.	37
(Stokely-Van Camp) stewed	½ cup	35
(Van Camp) whole	½ cup	25
Canned, dietetic pack:		
(Diet Delight)	½ cup	25
(Featherweight)	½ cup	20
(S&W) *Nutradiet,* whole	½ cup	25

Food and Description	Measure or Quantity	Calories
TOMATO JUICE:		
Canned, regular pack:		
(Campbell)	6-fl.-oz. can	35
(Del Monte)	6-fl.-oz. can	36
(Libby's)	6-fl.-oz. can	35
Musselman's	6 fl. oz.	30
Canned, dietetic pack:		
(Diet Delight)	6 fl. oz.	35
(Featherweight)	6 fl. oz.	35
TOMATO JUICE COCKTAIL:		
(Ocean Spray) Firehouse Jubilee	6 fl. oz.	44
Snap-E-Tom	6 fl. oz.	40
TOMATO PASTE, canned:		
Regular pack:		
(Contadina) Italian	6 oz.	210
(Del Monte)	6-oz. can	163
(Hunt's)	6-oz. can	140
Dietetic (Featherweight) low sodium	6-oz. can	150
TOMATO & PEPPER, HOT CHILI		
(Ortega) Jalapeno	1-oz. serving	7
TOMATO, PICKLED (Claussen)		
green	1 piece	6
TOMATO PUREE, canned:		
Regular (Contadina) heavy	1 cup	100
Dietetic (Featherweight)	1 cup	90
TOMATO SAUCE, canned:		
(Contadina) regular	1 cup	90
(Del Monte):		
Regular	1 cup	86
Hot	1 cup	80
With tomato tidbits	1 cup	92
(Hunt's) with cheese	4-oz. serving	70
TOM COLLINS, canned (Mr. Boston)		
12½% alcohol	3 fl. oz.	105
TONGUE, beef, braised	4-oz. serving	277
TOPPING:		
Regular:		
Butterscotch (Smucker's)	1 T.	70
Caramel (Smucker's)	1 T.	70
Chocolate fudge (Hershey's)	1 T.	49
Pecans in syrup (Smucker's)	1 T.	65
Pineapple (Smucker's)	1 T.	65
Dietetic, chocolate (Diet Delight)	1 T.	16
TOPPING, WHIPPED:		
Regular:		
Cool Whip (Birds Eye), dairy	1 T.	16
Lucky Whip, aerosol	1 T.	12
Whip Topping (Rich's)	¼ oz.	20

Food and Description	Measure or Quantity	Calories
Dietetic (Featherweight)	1 T.	3
*Mix:		
Regular, *Dream Whip*	1 T.	5
Dietetic (D-Zerta)	1 T.	7
TOP RAMEN, beef (Nissin Foods)	3-oz. serving	390
TORTILLA (Amigos)	6″ × ⅛″ tortilla	111
TOSTADA, frozen (Van de Kamp's)	8½ oz.	530
TOSTADA SHELL (Ortega)	1 shell	50
TOTAL, cereal	1 cup	110
TRIPE, canned (Libby's)	6-oz. serving	290
TRIPLE SEC LIQUEUR		
(Mr. Boston)	1 fl. oz.	79
TRIX, cereal (General Mills)	1 cup	110
TUNA:		
Canned in oil:		
(Bumble Bee):		
Chunk, light, drained	6½-oz. can	309
Solids, white, drained	7-oz. can	333
(Carnation) solids & liq.	6½-oz. can	427
(Star Kist) solids, white, solids & liq.	7-oz. serving	503
Canned in water:		
(Breast O' Chicken)	6½-oz. can	211
(Bumble Bee):		
Chunk, light, solids & liq.	6½-oz. can	234
Solid, white, solids & liq.	7-oz. can	252
(Featherweight) light, chunk	6 ½ oz.	210
(Star Kist) light	7-oz. can	220
*TUNA HELPER** (General Mills):		
Country dumplings or noodles/cheese	⅕ of pkg.	230
Creamy noodle	⅕ of pkg.	280
TUNA PIE, frozen:		
(Banquet)	8-oz. pie	434
(Morton)	8-oz. pie	373
TUNA SALAD:		
Home recipe	4-oz. serving	193
Canned (Carnation)	¼ of 7½-oz. can	98
TURKEY:		
Barbecued (Louis Rich) breast, half	1 oz.	40
Canned:		
(Hormel) chunk	6¾-oz. serving	223
(Swanson) chunk	2½-oz. serving	120
Packaged:		
(Eckrich) sliced	1-oz. serving	47
(Hormel) breast	.8-oz. slice	29
(Louis Rich):		
Turkey bologna	1-oz. slice	60
Turkey cotto salami	1-oz. slice	50

Food and Description	Measure or Quantity	Calories
Turkey ham, chopped	1-oz. slice	45
Turkey pastrami	1-oz. slice	35
(Oscar Mayer) breast	¾-oz. slice	21
Roasted:		
Flesh & skin	4-oz. serving	253
Dark meat	2½″ × 1⅝″ × ¼″ slice	43
Light meat	4″ × 2″ × ¼″ slice	75
Smoked (Louis Rich):		
Drumsticks	1 oz. (without bone)	40
Wing drumettes	1 oz. (without bone)	45
TURKEY DINNER OR ENTREE, frozen:		
(Banquet):		
Regular	11-oz. dinner	293
Man Pleaser	19-oz. dinner	620
(Green Giant)	9-oz. entree	404
(Swanson):		
Regular, with gravy & dressing	9¼-oz. entree	310
Hungry Man	18¾-oz. dinner	600
TV Brand	11½-oz. dinner	340
(Weight Watchers) sliced, 3-compartment	15¼-oz. meal	390
TURKEY PIE, frozen:		
(Banquet):		
Regular	8-oz. pie	415
Supreme	8-oz. pie	430
(Morton)	8-oz. pie	334
(Stouffer's)	10-oz. pie	460
(Swanson):		
Regular	8-oz. pie	430
Hungry Man	1-lb. pie	730
TURKEY TETRAZINI, frozen:		
(Stouffer's)	6-oz. serving	240
(Weight Watchers)	13-oz. bag	403
TUMERIC (French's)	1 tsp.	7
TURNIP GREENS, canned (Sunshine) chopped, solids & liq.	½ cup	19
TURNOVER:		
Frozen (Pepperidge Farm):		
Apple or cherry	1 turnover	310
Blueberry, peach or raspberry	1 turnover	320
Refrigerated (Pillsbury):		
Apple or blueberry	1 turnover	170
Cherry	1 turnover	180
TWINKIE (Hostess):		
Regular	1 cake	155
Devil's food	1 cake	150

Food and Description	Measure or Quantity	Calories

V

Food and Description	Measure or Quantity	Calories
VALPOLICELLA WINE (Antinori)	3 fl. oz.	84
VANDERMINT, liqueur	1 fl. oz.	90
VANILLA EXTRACT (Virginia Dare)	1 tsp.	10
VEAL, broiled, medium cooked:		
Loin chop	4 oz.	265
Rib, roasted	4 oz.	305
Steak or cutlet, lean & fat	4 oz.	245
VEAL DINNER, frozen:		
(Banquet) parmigiana	11-oz. dinner	421
(Swanson):		
Hungry Man, parmigiana	20½-oz. dinner	700
TV Brand, parmigiana	12¼-oz. dinner	450
(Weight Watchers) parmigiana, 2-compartment	9-oz. meal	243
VEAL STEAK, frozen (Hormel):		
Regular	4-oz. serving	131
Breaded	4-oz. serving	242
VEGETABLE BOUILLON (Herb-Ox):		
Cube	1 cube	6
Packet	1 packet	12
VEGETABLE JUICE COCKTAIL:		
Regular, *V-8*	6 fl. oz.	35
Dietetic:		
(Featherweight)	6 fl. oz.	35
(S&W) *Nutradiet,* low sodium	6 fl. oz.	35
V-8, low sodium	6 fl. oz.	40
VEGETABLES, MIXED:		
Canned, regular pack:		
(Del Monte) drained	½ cup	51
(La Choy):		
Chinese	1 cup	24
Chop Suey	1 cup	36
(Libby's) solids & liq.	½ cup	40
Canned, dietetic pack (Featherweight)	½ cup	40
Frozen:		
(Birds Eye):		
Regular:		
Broccoli, cauliflower & carrots in cheese sauce	3⅓ oz.	90
Carrots, peas & onions, deluxe	3⅓ oz.	52

Food and Description	Measure or Quantity	Calories
Mixed, with onion sauce	2.7 oz.	110
Pea & pearl onion	3⅓ oz.	92
Pea & potato with cream sauce	2.7 oz.	164
Stew	6.7 oz.	103
Blue Ribbon:		
Broccoli, carrots & pasta in lightly seasoned sauce	3⅓ oz.	92
Corn, green beans & pasta in lightly seasoned sauce	3⅓ oz.	115
Farm Fresh:		
Broccoli, cauliflower & carrot strips	3.2 oz.	30
Broccoli, corn & red pepper	3.2 oz.	58
Brussels sprouts, cauliflower & carrots	3.2 oz.	36
International Style:		
Chinese style	3⅓ oz.	85
Italian style	3⅓ oz.	130
Japanese style	3⅓ oz.	102
Mexican style	3⅓ oz.	133
Stir Fry:		
Cantonese style	⅓ of pkg.	56
Chinese style	⅓ of pkg.	36
Japanese style	⅓ of pkg.	32
(Green Giant):		
Regular:		
Broccoli, cauliflower & carrots in cheese sauce	3⅓ oz.	55
Mixed	3⅓ oz.	60
Harvest Fresh	4 oz.	68
Harvest Get Together:		
Broccoli-cauliflower medley	3⅓ oz.	50
Broccoli fanfare	3⅓ oz.	66
Japanese style	3⅓ oz.	38
(Le Seuer) peas, onions & carrots in butter sauce	3⅓ oz.	72
(La Choy):		
Chinese	5-oz. serving	36
Japanese	5-oz. serving	36
(McKenzie)	3⅓ oz.	65
(Southland):		
California blend	⅕ of 16-oz. pkg.	35
Oriental	⅕ of 16-oz. pkg.	30
Stew	4 oz.	60
VEGETABLES IN PASTRY, frozen (Pepperidge Farm):		
Asparagus with mornay sauce or broccoli with cheese	3¾ oz.	250

139

Food and Description	Measure or Quantity	Calories
Cauliflower & cheese sauce	3¾ oz.	220
Spinach almondine	3¾ oz.	260
Zucchini provencal	3¾ oz.	210
VEGETABLE STEW, canned, *Dinty Moore*	7½-oz. serving	163
"VEGETARIAN FOODS":		
Canned or dry:		
Chicken, fried (Loma Linda) with gravy	1½-oz. piece	109
Chili (Worthington)	¼ can (5-oz. serving)	190
Choplet (Worthington)	1 choplet	50
Dinner cuts (Loma Linda) drained	1 cut	54
Franks, big (Loma Linda)	1.9-oz. frank	100
Franks, sizzle (Loma Linda)	2.2-oz. frank	167
FriChik (Worthington)	1 piece	95
Granburger (Worthington)	6 T.	130
Little links (Loma Linda) drained	.8-oz. link	45
Non-meatballs (Worthington)	1 meatball	165
Nuteena (Loma Linda)	½" slice	165
Proteena (Loma Linda)	½" slice	144
Sandwich spread:		
(Loma Linda)	1 T.	24
(Worthington)	2½ oz.	120
Savorex (Loma Linda)	1 T.	32
Soyagen, all-purpose powder (Loma Linda)	1 T.	48
Soyalac (Loma Linda):		
I-soyalac	1 cup	177
Concentrate, liquid	1 cup	351
Ready to use	1 cup	166
Soyameat (Worthington):		
Sliced beef	1 slice	55
Diced chicken	¼ cup	120
Sliced chicken	1 slice	65
Salisbury steak	1 slice	160
Soyamel, any kind (Worthington)	1 oz.	145
Stew pack (Loma Linda) drained	1 piece	7
Super links (Worthington)	1 link	120
Swiss steak with gravy (Loma Linda)	1 steak	138
Tender bits (Loma Linda) drained	1 piece	23
Vege-burger (Loma Linda) no salt added	½ cup	119
Vegelona (Loma Linda)	½" slice	102
Vega-Links (Worthington)	1 link	70
Wheat protein	4 oz.	124
Worthington 209	1 slice	75

Food and Description	Measure or Quantity	Calories
Frozen:		
Beef-like slices (Worthington)	1 slice	60
Beef pie (Worthington)	1 pie	470
Bologna (Loma Linda)	1 oz.	77
Chicken (Loma Linda)	1 slice	57
Chicken, fried (Loma Linda)	2-oz. serving	188
Chicken pie (Worthington)	1 pie	450
Chic-Ketts (Worthington)	½ cup	180
Corned beef, loaf, or sliced (Worthington)	2½ oz.	190
FriPats (Worthington)	1 pat	180
Meatballs (Loma Linda)	1 meatball	46
Prosage (Worthington)	1 link	60
Roast Beef (Loma Linda)	1 oz.	65
Sausage, breakfast (Loma Linda)	⅓" slice	72
Smoked beef, roll (Worthington)	2½ oz.	170
Turkey (Loma Linda)	1 oz.	61
Wham, roll (Worthington)	2½ oz.	140
VERMOUTH:		
Dry & extra dry (Lejon; Noilly Pratt)	1 fl. oz.	33
Sweet (Lejon; Taylor)	1 fl. oz.	45
VICHY WATER (Schweppes)	Any quantity	0
VIENNA SAUSAGE:		
(Hormel):		
Regular	1 sausage	53
Chicken	1-oz. serving	60
(Libby's):		
In barbecue sauce	2½ oz.	180
In beef broth	1 link	46
VINEGAR	1 T.	2

W

WAFFELOS, cereal (Ralston Purina)	1 cup	110
WAFFLE, frozen:		
(Aunt Jemima) jumbo	1 waffle	86
(Eggo):		
Blueberry or strawberry	1 waffle	130
Home style	1 waffle	120
WALNUT, English or Persian (Diamond A)	1 cup	679
WALNUT FLAVORING, Black (Durkee) imitation	1 tsp.	4

Food and Description	Measure or Quantity	Calories
WATER CHESTNUT, canned:		
(Chun King) solids & liq.	8½-oz. can	140
(La Choy) drained	¼ of 8-oz. can	16
WATERCRESS, trimmed	½ cup	3
WATERMELON:		
Wedge	4″ × 8″ wedge	111
Diced	½ cup	21
WELSH RAREBIT:		
Home recipe	1 cup	415
Frozen:		
(Green Giant)	5-oz. serving	219
(Stouffer's)	5-oz. serving	355
WESTERN DINNER, frozen:		
(Banquet)	11-oz. dinner	417
(Morton) *Round-Up*	11.8-oz. dinner	426
(Swanson):		
Hungry Man	17¾-oz. dinner	820
TV Brand	11¾-oz. dinner	430
WHEATENA, cereal	¼ cup	112
WHEAT FLAKES CEREAL:		
(Breakfast Best)	1 cup	141
(Featherweight)	1¼ cups	100
(Van Brode)	¾ cup	106
WHEAT GERM, RAW (Elam's)	1 oz.	112
WHEAT GERM CEREAL		
(Kretschmer):		
Regular	¼ cup	99
Brown sugar & honey	¼ cup	114
WHEAT HEARTS, cereal (General Mills)	1 oz.	110
WHEATIES, cereal	1 cup	110
WHEAT & OATMEAL, cereal, hot (Elam's)	1 oz.	105
WHISKEY SOUR COCKTAIL, canned (Mr. Boston)	3 fl. oz.	120
WHITE CASTLE:		
Bun	.8 oz.	65
Cheeseburger (meat & cheese only)	1.54-oz. serving	120
Fish sandwich (fish only, without tartar sauce)	1.48-oz. serving	127
French fries	2.6-oz. serving	225
Hamburger (meat only, no bun)	1.2-oz. serving	95
WHITEFISH, LAKE:		
Baked, stuffed	4 oz.	244
Smoked	4 oz.	176
WILD BERRY DRINK, canned (Hi-C)	6 fl. oz.	88

Food and Description	Measure or Quantity	Calories
WINCHELL'S DONUT HOUSE:		
Buttermilk, old fashioned	2-oz. piece	249
Cake, devil's food, iced	2-oz. piece	241
Cinnamon crumb	2-oz. piece	240
Iced, chocolate	2-oz. piece	227
Raised, glazed	1¾-oz. piece	212
WINE, COOKING (Regina):		
Burgundy or sauterne	¼ cup	2
Sherry	¼ cup	20

Y

Food and Description	Measure or Quantity	Calories
YEAST, BAKER'S (Fleischmann's):		
Dry, active	¼ oz.	20
Fresh & household, active	.6-oz. cake	15
YOGURT:		
Regular:		
Plain:		
(Bison)	8-oz. container	160
(Colombo):		
Regular	8-oz. container	150
Natural Lite	8-oz. container	110
(Dannon)	8-oz. container	150
(Friendship)	8-oz. container	170
Yoplait	6-oz. container	130
Plain with honey, *Yoplait, Custard Style*	6-oz. container	160
Apple:		
(Colombo) spiced	8-oz. container	240
(Dannon) Dutch	8-oz. container	260
Mélangé	6-oz. container	180
Yoplait (General Mills)	6-oz. container	190
Apple-cinnamon, *Yoplait, Breakfast Yogurt*	6-oz. container	240
Apricot (Bison)	8-oz. container	262
Banana:		
(Dannon)	8-oz. container	260
LeShake (Kellogg)	8-oz. container	170
Banana-strawberry (Colombo)	8-oz. container	235
Berry (New Country) mixed	8-oz. container	210
Blueberry:		
(Bison):		
Regular	8-oz. container	262
Light	6-oz. container	162
(Colombo)	8-oz. container	250

Food and Description	Measure or Quantity	Calories
(Dannon)	8-oz. container	260
(Friendship)	8-oz. container	230
Mélangé	6-oz. container	180
(New Country) supreme	8-oz. container	210
(Sweet'n Low)	8-oz. container	150
Yoplait (General Mills)	6-oz. container	190
Boysenberry:		
(Bison)	8-oz. container	262
(Dannon)	8-oz. container	260
(Sweet'n Low)	8-oz. container	150
Cherry:		
(Bison) light	6-oz. container	162
(Colombo) black	8-oz. container	230
(Dannon)	8-oz. container	260
(Friendship)	8-oz. container	230
Mélangé	6-oz. container	180
(Sweet'n Low)	8-oz. container	150
Yoplait	6-oz. container	190
Cherry-vanilla (Colombo)	8-oz. container	250
Citrus, *Yoplait, Breakfast Yogurt*	6-oz. container	250
Coffee (Colombo; Dannon)	8-oz. container	200
Coffee, *Yoplait, Custard Style*	6-oz. container	180
Date-Walnut-Raisin (Bison)	8-oz. container	262
Fruit Crunch (New Country)	8-oz. container	210
Granola strawberry (Colombo)	8-oz. container	240
Guava (Colombo)	8-oz. container	240
Hawaiian salad (New Country)	8-oz. container	210
Honey vanilla (Colombo)	8-oz. container	220
Lemon:		
(Dannon)	8-oz. container	200
(Sweet'N Low)	8-oz. container	150
Yoplait:		
Regular	6-oz. container	190
Custard Style	6-oz. container	180
Orange, *Yoplait*	6-oz. container	190
Orange supreme (New Country)	8-oz. container	210
Orchard, *Yoplait, Breakfast Yogurt*	6-oz. container	240
Peach:		
(Bison)	8-oz. container	262
(Dannon)	8-oz. container	260
(Friendship)	8-oz. container	230
(New Country) 'n cream	8-oz. container	240
(Sweet'N Low)	8-oz. container	150
Peach melba (Colombo)	8-oz. container	230
Piña Colada:		
(Colombo)	8-oz. container	240
(Dannon)	8-oz. container	260
(Friendship)	8-oz. container	230

Food and Description	Measure or Quantity	Calories
Pineapple:		
(Bison) light	6-oz. container	162
Mélangé	6-oz. container	180
Raspberry:		
(Colombo)	8-oz. container	250
(Dannon) red	8-oz. container	260
(Friendship)	8-oz. container	230
Mélangé (Dannon)	6-oz. container	180
(Sweet'N Low)	8-oz. container	150
Yoplait	6-oz. container	190
Yoplait, Custard Style	6-oz. container	180
Raspberry ripple (New Country)	8-oz. container	240
Strawberry:		
(Bison) light	6-oz. container	162
(Colombo)	8-oz. container	230
(Dannon)	8-oz. container	260
(Friendship)	8-oz. container	230
Mélangé	6-oz. container	180
(Sweet'N Low)	8-oz. container	150
Yoplait	6-oz. container	190
Strawberry banana (Sweet'N Low)	8-oz. container	150
Strawberry colada (Colombo)	8-oz. container	230
Tropical fruit (Sweet'N Low)	8-oz. container	150
Vanilla:		
(Dannon)	8-oz. container	200
(New Country) French, ripple	8-oz. container	240
Yoplait, Custard Style	6-oz. container	180
Frozen, hard:		
Banana:		
Danny-Yo	3½-oz. serving	110
Danny-in-a-Cup	8-oz. cup	210
Boysenberry:		
Danny-On-A-Stick, carob coated	2½-fl.-oz. bar	135
Danny-Yo	3½-oz. serving	110
Boysenberry swirl (Bison)	¼ of 16-oz. container	116
Cherry vanilla (Bison)	¼ of 16-oz. container	116
Chocolate:		
(Bison)	¼ of 16-oz. container	116
(Colombo) bar, chocolate coated	1 bar	145
(Dannon):		
Danny-in-a-Cup	8-fl. oz. cup	210
Danny-On-A-Stick, chocolate coated	2½-fl. oz. bar	135
Chocolate chip (Bison)	¼ of 16-oz. container	116
Chocolate chocolate chip (Colombo)	4-oz. serving	150
Mocha (Colombo) bar	1 bar	80

Food and Description	Measure or Quantity	Calories
Pina Colada:		
(Colombo)	4-oz. serving	110
(Dannon):		
Danny-in-a-Cup	8-oz. cup	210
Danny-On-A-Stick	2½-fl.-oz. bar	65
Raspberry, red (Dannon)		
Danny-On-A-Stick, chocolate coated	2½-fl.-oz. bar	135
Danny-in-a-Cup	8-oz. container	210
Danny-Yo	3½-fl. oz.	110
Raspberry swirl (Bison)	¼ of 16-oz. container	116
Strawberry:		
(Bison)	¼ of 16-oz. container	116
(Colombo):		
Regular	4-oz. serving	110
Bar	1 bar	80
(Dannon):		
Danny-in-a-Cup	8 fl. oz.	210
Danny-Yo	3½ fl. oz.	110
Vanilla:		
(Bison)	¼ of 16-oz. container	116
(Colombo):		
Regular	4-oz. serving	110
Bar, chocolate covered	1 bar	145
(Dannon):		
Danny-in-a-Cup	8 fl. oz.	180
Danny-On-A-Stick	2½-fl.-oz. bar	65
Danny-Yo	3½-oz. serving	110
Frozen, soft (Colombo)	6-fl.-oz. serving	130

Z

ZINFANDEL WINE (Inglenook)		
Vintage	3 fl. oz.	59
ZITI, frozen (Weight Watchers)	12½-oz. pkg.	342
ZWIEBACK (Gerber; Nabisco)	1 piece	30